THE

HERBAL
HOME SPA

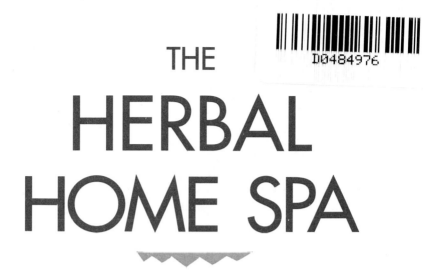

NATURALLY REFRESHING WRAPS, RUBS, LOTIONS, MASKS, OILS, AND SCRUBS

GRETA BREEDLOVE

STOREY

Storey Books
Schoolhouse Road
Pownal, Vermont 05261

The mission of Storey Communications is to serve our customers
by publishing practical information that encourages
personal independence in harmony with the environment.

Edited by Deborah L. Balmuth
Cover illustration by Laura Tedeschi
Cover and text design and production by Susan Bernier (based on an original
    design by Carol Jessop, Black Trout Design)
Line drawings by Sarah Brill (p. 66, 153), Judy Eliason (p. 10), Brigita
    Fuhrmann (p. 56, 80), Alison Kolesar (p. 46), Randy Mosher (p. 4, 45,
    47, 49, 50, 51, 58, 84, 100, 117, 149, 152), Frank Riccio (p. 136, 137), and
    Laura Tedeschi (p. 54, 68, 72, 74, 87, 89, 91, 93, 109, 110, 112, 123, 127,
    145, 150, 163)
Indexed by Randl W. Ockey
Professional assistance by Wendy Liebenow

The information in this book is true and complete to the best of our knowledge.
All recommendations are made without guarantee on the part of the author or
Storey Communications, Inc. The author and publisher disclaim any liability in con-
nection with the use of this information. For additional information please contact
Storey Communications, Inc., Schoolhouse Road, Pownal, Vermont 05261.

Storey Publishing books are available for special premium and promotional
uses and for customized editions. For further information, please call the Custom
Publishing Department at 800-793-9396.

Printed in the United States by R.R. Donnelley
10 9 8 7 6 5 4 3 2 1

Library of Congress Cataloging-in-Publication Data

Breedlove, Greta
    The herbal home spa : naturally refreshing wraps, rubs, lotions, masks, oils,
and scrubs / Greta Breedlove.
        p.   cm.
    ISBN 1-58017-005-6 (pbk. : alk. paper)
    1. Beauty, Personal.   2. Herbal cosmetics.   3. Women—Health and hygiene.
    I. Title.
RA778.G34   1998
646.7'2—dc21   97-44761
                                                                                         CIP

DEDICATION

For my mother, Jean Marie Breedlove, who brought me into this world and cared for and nurtured me. Whose Spirit believed that nothing that is creative is a mess and so instilled, nurtured, and nourished my creativity. Thanks, Mom.

And for my sisters, Jeanne Litt, Anne Breedlove Eldredge, and Mary Breedlove Gray.

Jeanne, who while in nursing school would bathe me as a little girl with her tenderness and a fun way to wrap the washcloth.

Anne, who in her wild spirit snuck me up to my mother's bedroom to pierce my ears when I was six and also used to talk to Trees!

Mary, whose creativity resulted in endless buns in my hair for dance recitals and a scary witch on more than one Halloween.

And for all women, give yourselves permission to take the time to do the things that nourish your soul, honor the goddess within, and cherish the feminine in all things.

ACKNOWLEDGMENTS

Special thanks to the following: Chatham Public Library staff; Pamela Lappies, courier extraordinaire; Michael Schaffer, Joel Feldman, Kathleen Palladino, for helping me keep my body, mind, and Spirit in balance during the process of writing this book; Charles Kleinbaum, Mary Zander, Nancy Litt, for helpful guidance; James Eldredge, Barry Litt, Ann Eldredge, for technical assistance; Scott Garber and Arthur Breedlove for research assistance; all the herbal authors and teachers who have gone before me, especially those listed in the bibliography; Peace Theology Seminary Master's Program; University of Santa Monica; John Roger, John Morton, and the Movement of Spiritual Inner Awareness; the Storey staff who worked on this book; and Deborah Balmuth, my talented editor, who truly made this book possible. Thank you.

And thanks to Scott Garber, my dear husband, partner, and best friend. We made it!

TABLE OF CONTENTS

PREFACE

Looking and feeling your most beautiful means pampering all of you. It takes a total approach, encompassing mind, body, and spirit, to be truly healthy and glowing. Simply setting aside time for yourself is a big step in the right direction.

What you do with that time can vary. I've always been drawn to the pampering treatments that luxury spas offer, yet my budget won't allow the frequent visits I might like. So I set out to demystify these treatments and create the same indulgences at home.

Growing up in a large family with a do-it-yourself mom, I knew I could create recipes similar to those available in salons. Being sensitive to many commercial products, my skin and something deep within me craved simple, natural products and their gentle care.

Early on in my formal training as an herbalist apprenticing with Pam Montgomery, Pam encouraged me to expand on my natural inclination toward creating body care products. I began to read and experiment with recipes. Rosemary Gladstar's *Natural Skin and Body Care* got me started. I also made it a point to "pick the brains" of the staff at the salons and spas that I visited.

One unexpected aspect I discovered as I worked in body care was the satisfaction that comes from nurturing oneself. No esthetician, masseuse, or salon worker can foster your sense of well-being in quite the way that giving to yourself lovingly can.

And so this call was more than just a delving into creating herbal body treatments. It was a call to the glorification of all that is feminine in me and others, even men; a celebration of the nurturer, the tender spirit, the divine caregiver. As much as the feminist movement has done to open doors for women, there is still much devaluing of the feminine in our culture. This book is full of "rituals" for valuing the divine goddess in each of you.

With the creation of herbal treatments, a relationship as old as the beginning of time is also honored and renewed. This relationship with our green friends and the healing gifts they offer to us in the form of herbs, flowers, trees, and fragrances is a relationship offering peace. My hope and my wish for you is a greater connection first to yourself, then of course to others and this wonderful planet of ours. Green Blessings.

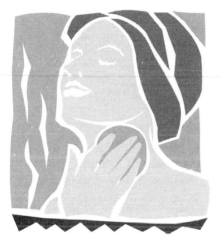

The Natural Approach to a Beautiful Body

CHAPTER 1

There are a lot of good reasons to make your own skin-care products. Many people are opting for a natural approach to lifestyle, from dietary choices to skin-care products. By making your own treatments, you can be sure of exactly what goes into them. Some of you, like me, may have experienced allergic reactions to many commercial skin-care products and seek natural products out of necessity. Maybe you feel that commercial skin-care products are too expensive and you just don't want to pay the high prices. You may have received a treatment at a salon and thought, "I can do this myself at home." And you're right; there are many treatments that you can do for yourself at home for a fraction of the cost of a salon visit.

HEAD-TO-TOE TREATMENTS

Beginning with the head and face and working our way down the body with treatments for the full torso, the hands, and finally the feet, you'll find pampering here for every part of the body. In the final chapter, I suggest some ways to create treatment routines that work well as part of your regular self-care. I also encourage you to share these relaxing treatments with friends and loved ones.

Before introducing you to the ingredients, supplies, and simple equipment you'll need, I would like to encourage you to think about the ideas in this book as part of a larger whole — your health and well-being. Radiant, healthy skin is a result of many factors: a healthy diet, plenty of exercise, good skin-care practices, and a positive, relaxed mental attitude.

ADOPTING A LIFESTYLE FOR RADIANT SKIN

A healthy diet is essential to radiant skin. There is so much information available on diets to keep you healthy that I cannot even begin to scratch the surface in this book. However, I will stress that you need to consume plenty of fresh fruits and vegetables every day. (No, potato chips do not qualify as a vegetable!) If you don't like fruits and vegetables, experiment with preparing them in various ways until you find some that you enjoy. Eating a balanced and varied diet is important.

Drink Plenty of Water

Water is crucial for healthy skin, helping to keep it soft and supple. Many of the recipes in this book use water to cleanse the skin externally; but it is even more beneficial when consumed internally. Doctors recommend drinking eight 8-ounce glasses of water each day, and more if you are sick or out in the sun or heat. You will get much better results from your skin-care products and treatments if you consume the recommended amounts of water. One of the side benefits of drinking plenty of water is that it is also helpful if you are trying to lose weight.

Nourish Your Skin with Herbal Teas

Another way to help hydrate the skin and receive vitamins and minerals important to overall health is by drinking herbal teas. They are easy to make and there are any number of different teas to choose from. I like to purchase the loose herbs for making teas (often available in bulk at natural and specialty food stores) rather than tea bags because I can better judge the freshness of the herbs. If you don't have a choice, tea from tea bags is still a good, healthy alternative to soft drinks. Do some tea tasting to see which herbs you like best, and try combining several. If you find a commercial tea-bag combination you like, look at the list of ingredients and try creating your own version. While almost any herbs are good for you, I've listed a few that are particularly nourishing for the skin and hair.

Mixing herbal tea with fruit juice is a great way to get natural sweetness and the benefits of the herbs at the same time. If you are making a juice from concentrate, try using herbal tea in place of the water portion. I usually like to add a little more water as well, because most commercial juices are too sweet for me.

HERBS FOR SKIN AND HAIR

- Black alder (for skin eruptions)
- Bergamot tea (cleanses the system)
- Burdock
- Dandelion
- Horsetail
- Nettles
- Oat straw
- Sarsaparilla
- Stevia
- Yellow dock

BREWED HERBAL TEA

1 tablespoon (15 ml) fresh herbs (1 teaspoon [5 ml] dried) for each 8 ounces (227 g) of water

To make: Bring water to a boil. Put the herbs in a heatproof glass jar (such as a Mason jar); pour the boiling water over herbs and cover. Allow flowers to steep for 5 minutes; leafy materials should steep for 20 minutes to 4 hours. The longer the steeping time, the more medicinal the tea. Strain out herbs and discard (or add to the compost pile).

To use: Drink 3 cups per day.

Exercise, Relax, and Receive with Joy

Regular exercise promotes good blood circulation, which in turn helps maintain healthy skin. Find a form of exercise that you enjoy and schedule it into your daily routine. Exercise also helps relieve stress and promotes a healthy mental attitude, another element in achieving radiant skin.

Relaxation is key to enjoying and getting the most from these herbal treatments. Herbs, flowers, and the other natural ingredients are God's gifts to each of us. When you're ready to use these formulas, set aside the time and space to allow yourself to truly receive these natural gifts and experience the wonder of their healing powers.

Most important of all, have fun making these products. Let yourself become absorbed in the creative process of making these treatment to nurture and nourish yourself. Put your love into your formulas. It makes a difference.

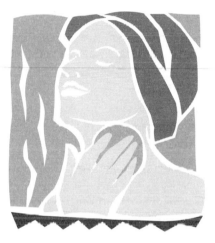

A Guide to Knowing and Selecting Natural Ingredients

CHAPTER 2

Learning to make your own skin-care products can save you a bundle of money, but don't skimp on the quality of the ingredients in your money-saving efforts. Using the best quality ingredients is a good practice. Unfortunately, it's not always easy to assess the quality of natural products such as herbs; price is not always the best indicator of quality.

PURCHASING HERBS

Many of the preparations in this book are best made with fresh herbs, especially the teas, infusions, facial masks, plasters, poultices, and body scrubs. But it is not always possible to obtain fresh herbs. You can substitute dried herbs for fresh and vice versa, if herbs are not available in the preferred form. One part dried is roughly equal to two parts fresh. Growing your own herbs is best, of course (see pages 7 to 11), but buying them locally is a good alternative. Some of the herbs used in these recipes are not grown locally, and you will have to purchase them.

Many health food stores carry a selection of dried herbs as well as the oils required to create your favorite products. There are a growing number of retail businesses selling herbal products. A great deal of herbal business is done through mail-order catalogs, but you may be surprised at the listing of shops you'll find in your local Yellow Pages. There are several organizations and publications you can consult to find herb businesses near you (see resource list).

What to Look For

In purchasing dried herbs, one of the primary indicators of freshness is color. Bright green nettles are preferable to those that are faded brown. Oat straw should be a chartreuse green color as opposed to yellow-tan. Shelf life for dried herbs is short, about one year for most. Try to purchase your herbs from a source that renews its supply of herbs often. Ask questions about freshness. It's worth it to pay a higher price for more vital and colorful dried herbs.

Buy Organic

One important quality to insist on when buying fruits, vegetables, herbs, seeds, and oils is that they be organic, which means they are free of unnecessary chemicals and pesticide residues. You'll find that this does make a difference. More and more grocery stores as well as specialty food shops are offering organic ingredients. If you live in an area where organic ingredients are not available, or you simply cannot afford the added expense, don't let that stand in the way of making your products. Use the best quality ingredients you can find, but be sure to ask your grocer to stock affordable organic ingredients. The more people ask for them, the more stores are likely to respond to this consumer demand.

GROWING YOUR OWN HERBS

What a rewarding endeavor it is to grow your own herbs. They are so wonderful to have around, beautifying your home and imparting their gentle aromas. Herbs from your own garden are the best possible ingredients for your finished products. An herb garden can range from a small kitchen window box to a large garden plot. Herbs have a variety of preferred growing conditions. Unlike vegetables, many herbs prefer poor soil. Growing your own herbs, then harvesting and drying them, is topic enough for a whole book. I offer a quick overview here, and encourage you to consult a few herb gardening books and try to re-create the native conditions for the plants you decide to grow (see bibliography).

Wildcrafting

Wildcrafting is the practice of harvesting plants from their natural habitat. Many useful plants grow abundantly in the wild and are offered by the Earth for the taking. Unfortunately, the recent herbal renaissance has not been good news for some plants. Although logging practices are often blamed for endangering many plant species, herbalists and wildcrafters have, in recent years, caused significant decline in populations of many plants that were gaining widespread interest.

In many places it is illegal to collect plants and even to pick a single flower. It is best to obtain permission to harvest on properties other than your own and to do so with respect for the land. Native American practice would have you speak to the plants, finding the Grandmother and asking permission to harvest. In their tradition, permission was received from the plants and seven plants were left untouched for the next seven generations. Harvesting was done from what was left. Imagine if our culture took on the philosophy of the Native Americans and preserved resources for the next seven generations, refraining from any practices that would bring harm to them as well.

WARNING: ASSESS THE DANGER FOR YOURSELF

Before you gather and use any plants from the wild, be sure you can identify those that are poisonous. We get quite alarmed when we hear the term poisonous, and rightly so. Unfortunately, the current warning system is confusing: All plants ever known to cause any ill effects regardless of dosage are labeled "poisonous" by the Food and Drug Administration (FDA). Herbs such as comfrey, which the FDA recommends not be used internally, is healing to the skin externally, yet it is included on lists of poisonous plants. Buttercups can cause stomach cramps and are labeled "poisonous," yet they are not nearly as dangerous as poison hemlock, which can cause death.

It is helpful to look further into why plants are labeled poisonous and what these plants will do and in which quantities. If a plant is thought to cause livestock to have photosensitivity when eaten in large quantities, is it best to regard that plant as poisonous and never use it? Some of these questions you will have to answer yourself.

I don't mean to minimize the danger of poisonous plants. Some plants can kill even the burliest of men in small doses. Other plants' ill effects have been overdramatized. We all like a good story.

It is important to remember that essential oils and some plants that seem benign — honey, for example — can cause serious problems for, and even death in, infants. Simply placing an essential oil container in its mouth, which a baby may do, can cause harm. Individuals with frailties or health conditions will need to be diligent in their research and careful in their use of plants.

Another common practice in wildcrafting to preserve endangered plants and protect other plants is to harvest only one-third or one-fourth of any stand. Unfortunately, this practice, while well intentioned, does not work with the increasing numbers of people wildcrafting, especially for plants like ginseng, goldenseal, and lady's slipper.

If you wish to collect your own plants in the wild, do learn to identify them correctly and which plants are endangered, threatened, and poisonous. Many plants that are endangered or threatened can be planted and grown in your own yard or garden, thus preserving their special healing properties for future generations. Learn the endangered plants in your area and forego harvesting them. For more information on endangered plants, contact United Plant Savers (see resource list).

HARVESTING HERBS AND FLOWERS

Timely harvesting and drying are most important when growing and using your own herbs. Living in the Northeast as I do, it is not always easy to dry herbs and obtain a quality product because of the humidity and showers that often occur at harvest time. Yet it is still worth the effort. Harvest your herbs and flowers just prior to the fullness of their bloom. The plants will continue to bloom for a few days after harvesting.

Harvest herbs and flowers from 9 A.M. to 11 A.M., before the sun gets too hot, but after the morning dew has evaporated. This preserves the quality of the herbs, keeping their aromatic oils and other properties at their greatest strength.

Use a sharp knife or a razor blade to cut the herbs. It is easiest for the herbs to regenerate and continue to grow if you cut the stem just above a node or a blade. Harvest only as much as you can hang or store immediately.

Drying Herbs and Flowers by Hanging

Long-stemmed herbs and flowers lend themselves to drying by hanging in bunches. Herbs such as lavender, mugwort, St.-John's-wort, peony, baby's breath, and borage, as well as any flowering-top herbs, dry well as hanging bundles. As much as possible, collect herbs in dry weather. Simply gather a bundle

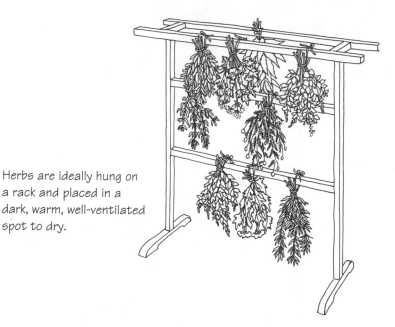

Herbs are ideally hung on a rack and placed in a dark, warm, well-ventilated spot to dry.

of herbs together, no more than about the thickness of your finger. I like to use rubber bands to secure the herbs because then they won't slip out; herbs shrink slightly when dry. I tie small pieces of string to the rubber band and hang the herbs in an area that is dark and well ventilated. Ideal drying temperature is between 65°F and 80°F.

Herbs and flowers can take anywhere from a few days to several weeks to dry. It is important to store herbs in dark, covered containers once they are dry, since a change in the humidity, such as a thunderstorm (where I live, common in July), can cause the herbs and flowers to absorb moisture and mold. Herbs and flowers should be dry and crisp, yet not so brittle as to break off.

Drying Herbs and Flowers on Screens

Wire screens are ideal for drying smaller herbs, leaves, and flowers, such as mints, rose petals, rosemary, violets, and violet leaf. You may use a well-cleaned old window screen free of lead paint or create your own by stretching screening or netting over a frame. Simply spread the herbs or flowers in a single layer on the screen, allowing air to circulate around the herbs. Drying time is usually quicker on a screen than by the bundle.

Store herbs in tightly fitted, dark, closed containers immediately once they are dry and crisp.

STORING NATURAL INGREDIENTS

Dried herbs and flowers should be kept in clean, airtight containers and stored in a dark, cool, and dry location. Light from any source as well as heat will rob the plants of their healing properties. Colored glass jars and bottles are helpful in protecting herbs. Store herbs on a bottom shelf; heat rises, so it will be cooler down there.

Seeds and nuts are best stored in the freezer. They can be purchased more economically in bulk, and they will last indefinitely.

OVERVIEW OF FLOWERS, HERBS, SPICES, AND TREES

The following list offers a quick overview of the ingredients used in the recipes in this book. You won't need them all at once, but it is worth browsing through this list and becoming familiar with it before you go out to buy the ingredients. Then, you can refer back to it as needed when you encounter an ingredient you haven't used before. Most herb stores will carry the following herbs and flowers, or they will be able to order them for you. If you have difficulty obtaining ingredients, check the mail order suppliers in the list of resources at the back of the book.

ACACIA (*ACACIA* SPP.)
Parts Used: Flowers
Cosmetic Properties: Demulcent, emollient
Grows: All over the world, especially southern France
Recipes: Herbal baths, facial steams

AGRIMONY (*AGRIMONIA EUPATORIA*)
Parts Used: Flowering tops, leaves
Cosmetic Properties: Soothes sore muscles, heals blemishes
Grows: Native to Europe, cultivated in much of the United States
Recipes: Herbal baths, facial masks

ALDER (*ALNUS* SPP.)

Parts Used: Bark
Cosmetic Properties: Soothes skin irritations and inflammations
Grows: Northeast United States and Canada
Recipes: Herbal skin tea

ALFALFA (*MEDICAGO SATIVA*)

Parts Used: Leaves, sprouts, seeds
Cosmetic Properties: Exfoliant, protein digester, good source of vitamins
Grows: Naturalized to most of North America
Recipes: Cuticle cream, facial mask, baths, creams, oils

COSMETIC TERMS

Alterative. Restores health.
Antifungal. Clears and counters fungal infections.
Anti-inflammatory. Reduces swelling.
Antimicrobial. Destroys or inhibits growth of microorganisms.
Antioxidant. Inhibits binding of oxygen.
Antiseptic. Cleansing; counters germs and other microorganisms.
Astringent. Causing skin tissue to contract or tighten.
Carminative. Aids digestion and promotes fresh breath.
Demulcent. Soothing or mollifying (softening, tempering).
Diaphoretic. Induces perspiration.
Diuretic. Increases urination.
Effervescent. Creates small bubbles of gas.
Emollient. Softening or soothing.
Exfoliant. A product that removes dead skin cells on surface of skin.
Humectant. Promotes retention of moisture.
Regenerative. Restores or revives tissue growth.
Rubefacient. Irritating to the skin; causing redness.

ALKANET ROOT (ANCHUSA OFFICINALIS)

Parts Used: Root
Cosmetic Properties: Emollient, colorant, sun protection
Grows: Wild from Maine south to New Jersey and west to Ohio and Michigan
Recipes: Lip balms, salves, hair and nail color

ALLSPICE (PIMENTA DIOICA)

Parts Used: Dried berries
Cosmetic Properties: Colorant, fragrant, mildly anesthetic, astringent
Grows: Tropical
Recipes: Perfumes, cologne, ointments, creams

ALOE VERA (ALOE BARBADENSIS)

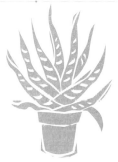

Parts Used: Gel from the leaves
Cosmetic Properties: Emollient, healing, soothes sunburns, regenerates damaged tissues
Grows: Native to Canary Islands; grow in pots almost anywhere but avoid cold; likes dry, sunny places and sandy soil
Recipes: Moisturizers, shampoos, skin creams

AMARANTH (AMARANTHUS HYBRIDUS)

Parts Used: Leaves, seeds
Cosmetic Properties: Regenerative, healing
Grows: Abundantly in vegetable gardens
Recipes: Wrinkle cream, eye cream

ANISE (PIMPINELLA ANISUM)

Parts Used: Seeds
Cosmetic Properties: Opens pores, fragrant, colorant
Grows: Cultivated throughout North America; occasionally found in the wild
Recipes: Hair rinses, scalp treatments

ARNICA (ARNICA MONTANA)

Parts Used: Flowers (*Note:* for external use only)
Cosmetic Properties: Stimulates hair growth, cures athlete's foot
Grows: Wild throughout North America
Recipes: Hair rinse

ARROWROOT (MARANTA ARUNDINACEA)

Parts Used: Tuberous rhizomes
Cosmetic Properties: Drying, powder base, demulcent
Grows: Americas, West Indies
Recipes: Foot and body powder

BALM OF GILEAD (POPULUS BALSAMIFERA)

Parts Used: Buds
Cosmetic Properties: Healing for sores, bruises, pimples, cuts
Grows: Central Appalachians west to Minnesota
Recipes: Burn and sunburn relief

BASIL (OCIMUM MINIMUM)

Parts Used: Leaves, essential oil
Cosmetic Properties: Hair growth and manageability
Grows: Annual cultivated in North America
Recipes: Scalp treatments, perfume

BAY (LAURUS NOBILIS); CALIFORNIA BAY (UMBELLULARIA CALIFORNICA)

Parts Used: Leaves
Cosmetic Properties: Stimulation, antiseptic, soothing
Grows: California
Recipes: Bay rum aftershave, facials, hair packs, herbal baths

BERGAMOT (MONARDA DIDYMA, M. PUNCTATA, M. FISTULOSA)

Parts Used: Tops, leaves
Cosmetic Properties: Rubefacient; as tea, cleanses system
Grows: Italy, France
Recipes: Facial masks and steams

TESTING FOR ALLERGIES

Even though an ingredient is natural, it may still provoke an allergic reaction in individuals prone to them. If you know you are allergic to specific herbs, fruits, nuts, or vegetables as food, it is best to avoid using these herbs topically as well.

If you are prone to allergic reactions, test ingredients on yourself with the following method:

1. Pour 1 teaspoon boiling water over ½ teaspoon of the dried herb, mixing to make a paste. Allow to cool.
2. Place paste on your inner arm, then cover with a bandage. Leave on until you react or for 24 hours. (Typical allergic reactions might be itching, redness, swelling, or irritation.)
3. Remove bandage. If there is a reaction, do not use the herb in future applications. To relieve any itchiness on the skin, make a paste of ground oats and place over the affected area. Oats are great for minor allergic skin reactions and itchy irritations. Occasionally, I have tested okay for an herb but still don't use it around the eye area, as my eyes are especially sensitive.

BIRCH (BETULA LENTA)
Parts Used: Bark
Cosmetic Properties: Fragrant, antiseptic, skin problems and eruptions
Grows: Northeastern United States and Canada
Recipes: Lotions, rinses, creams, baths

BLACKBERRY (RUBUS FRUTICOSUS)
Parts Used: Leaves, berries
Cosmetic Properties: Curative, astringent for blemishes and itchy skin
Grows: Wild or cultivated
Recipes: Herbal waters, skin freshener

BLACK MALVA (MALVA ROTUNDIFOLIA)
Parts Used: Flowers
Cosmetic Properties: Demulcent and emollient dye
Grows: Temperate zones
Recipes: Hair treatments

BLACK WALNUT (JUGLANS NIGRA)
Parts Used: Hulls, bark, leaves, oil
Cosmetic Properties: Astringent, antifungal
Grows: Temperate zones
Recipes: Mouthwash, douche, dye

BORAGE (BORAGO OFFICINALIS)
Parts Used: Flowering tops
Cosmetic Properties: Anti-inflammatory, demulcent,
emollient
Grows: Northeastern United States and Canada and south to
Tennessee and Illinois
Recipes: Facial masks

BURDOCK (ARCTIUM LAPPA)
Parts Used: Roots, leaves, seeds
Cosmetic Properties: Restorative for skin tone, smoothness;
for skin problems, astringent
Grows: Wild in northeastern United States and Canada
Recipes: Tea, facial steams, compresses

CALENDULA (CALENDULA OFFICINALIS)
Parts Used: Flowers
Cosmetic Properties: Accelerates healing, colorant
Grows: Easily in gardens
Recipes: Hair rinses, shampoos

CAYENNE (CAPSICUM ANNUUM VAR. ANNUUM)
Parts Used: Pepper pod powder
Cosmetic Properties: Stimulant, rubefacient, antiseptic
Grows: Cultivated in temperate North America
Recipes: Blemish treatments

CHAMOMILE (MATRICARIA RECUTITA)
Parts Used: Flowering tops, essential oil
Cosmetic Properties: Diaphoretic, restorative, mild
astringent
Grows: North America
Recipes: Facial masks and steams, eye cream, hair rinses

CHICKWEED (STELLARIA MEDIA)
Parts Used: Flowering top, leaves
Cosmetic Properties: Demulcent
Grows: Temperate North America
Recipes: Lotions, salves, bath

CINNAMON (CINNAMOMUM ZEYLANICUM)
Parts Used: Inner bark
Cosmetic Properties: Aromatic, astringent, fragrant
Grows: Tropical
Recipes: Hair rinses

CLARY SAGE (SALVIA SCLAREA)
Parts Used: Flowering tops, leaves, essential oil
Cosmetic Properties: Aromatic, astringent
Grows: Washington, Oregon, Kansas, Idaho
Recipes: Bath, lotions, hair products

CLEAVERS (GALIUM APARINE)
Parts Used: Aerial parts before flowering
Cosmetic Properties: Anti inflammatory, astringent
Grows: Wild throughout most of North America, Europe, and the Middle East
Recipes: Body-freshening tea

CLOVE (SYZYGIUM AROMATICUM)
Parts Used: Dried flower buds
Cosmetic Properties: Astringent, antiseptic, aromatic, colorant
Grows: Tropical
Recipes: Bath herb, hair rinse, waters, lotions

COLTSFOOT (TUSSILAGO FARFARA)
Parts Used: Leaves
Cosmetic Properties: Demulcent, emollient
Grows: Wild in northeastern United States and Canada
Recipes: Facial masks, steams

COMFREY *(SYMPHYTUM OFFICINALE)*
Parts Used: Leaves, root
Cosmetic Properties: Emollient, astringent, regenerates cells
Grows: Wild most everywhere
Recipes: Facial masks, steams, hair rinses, face creams

COWSLIP *(PRIMULA VERIS)*
Parts Used: Flower, leaves
Cosmetic Properties: Mild astringent, bleaching
Grows: Wild in temperate North America
Recipes: Hair products, facial scrubs, body powder

DANDELION (*TARAXACUM* SPP.)
Parts Used: Flower, leaves, root
Cosmetic Properties: Carminative; nourishing to liver, therefore good for skin eruptions and sensitivities
Grows: Wild throughout most of North America
Recipes: Facial steams, bath and body oils

DULSE *(PALMARIA PALMATA)*
Parts Used: Leaves
Cosmetic Properties: High mineral content, draws out impurities
Grows: Wild in North Atlantic salt water
Recipes: Thalassotherapy body wraps, herbal face lift

ECHINACEA *(ECHINACEA ANGUSTIFOLIA, ECHINACEA PURPUREA)*
Parts Used: Root, flower, powder
Cosmetic Properties: Antimicrobial
Grows: Wild in North America
Recipes: Blemish liniment

ELDER FLOWER *(SAMBUCUS CANADENSIS, S. NIGRA)*
Parts Used: Leaves, flowers, berries
Cosmetic Properties: Emollient, diaphoretic, gentle astringent
Grows: Wild in North America
Recipes: Face cream, bath and massage oil, sun products

ELM (*ULMUS* SPP.)
Parts Used: Bark, leaves
Cosmetic Properties: Astringent, emollient
Grows: Northeastern, central, and southeastern United States and Canada; other elms are found in Europe, Asia, and North Africa
Recipes: Facial masks

EUCALYPTUS (*EUCALYPTUS* SPP.)
Parts Used: Leaves, essential oil
Cosmetic Properties: Antiseptic, decongestant
Grows: Areas with average temperatures above 60°F
Recipes: Facial steams, scalp conditioner

EYEBRIGHT (*EUPHRASIA OFFICINALIS*)
Parts Used: Leaves, flowers
Cosmetic Properties: Astringent, anti-inflammatory
Grows: Wild and cultivated in North America
Recipes: Facial mask, eye cream

FENNEL (*FOENICULUM VULGARE*)
Parts Used: Seeds
Cosmetic Properties: Fragrant
Grows: Wild throughout the United States; originally a Mediterranean plant
Recipes: Facial steams, breath mints

FENUGREEK (*TRIGONELLA FOENUM-GRAECUM*)
Parts Used: Seeds
Cosmetic Properties: Skin softening
Grows: North America
Recipes: Facial masks

FEVERFEW (*CHRYSANTHEMUM PARTHENIUM*)
Parts Used: Flowers
Cosmetic Properties: Soothing to sensitive skin
Grows: Throughout the United States and southern Canada
Recipes: Bath herb, facial steam

FLAX *(LINUM USITATISSIMUM)*
Parts Used: Seeds
Cosmetic Properties: Emollient, demulcent
Recipes: Hair-setting gel, facial masks

GINGER *(ZINGIBER OFFICINALE)*
Parts Used: Root
Cosmetic Properties: Antiseptic
Recipes: Mouthwash

GINSENG *(PANAX QUINQUEFOLIUS)*
Parts Used: Root
Cosmetic Properties: Skin rejuvenator
Recipes: Baths, facial masks, lotions

GOLDENROD *(SOLIDAGO ODORA)*
Parts Used: Flowers, leaves
Cosmetic Properties: Aromatic, astringent, stimulating
Grows: Northern and eastern North America
Recipes: Facial steams, shampoos, hair rinses

GOLDENSEAL *(HYDRASTIS CANADENSIS)*
Parts Used: Powdered root
Cosmetic Properties: Astringent, stimulant
Grows: Native to North America
Recipes: Blemish liniment

HENNA *(LAWSONIA INERMIS)*
Parts Used: Powdered root
Cosmetic Properties: Dye
Grows: Native to Egypt and the Middle East
Recipes: Hair and nail color

HOLLYHOCK *(ALCEA ROSEA)*
Parts Used: Flowering top
Cosmetic Properties: Emollient, colorant
Grows: Northeastern United States
Recipes: Hair rinse, herbal baths, facial masks

HORSETAIL *(EQUISETUM ARVENSE)*
Parts Used: Aerial stems
Cosmetic Properties: Astringent, toning
Grows: Wild in North America
Recipes: Nail creme

INDIGO *(INDIGOFERA TINCTORIA)*
Parts Used: Flowering top
Cosmetic Properties: Colorant
Grows: North America
Recipes: Hair rinse

JASMINE *(JASMINUM OFFICINALE)*
Parts Used: Flowers, essential oil
Cosmetic Properties: Emollient, calming, fragrant, antiseptic
Grows: France, Morocco
Recipes: Massage oil, bath, facial steams

JEWELWEED *(IMPATIENS CAPENSIS)*
Parts Used: Juice, flowering tops
Cosmetic Properties: Drying, colorant
Grows: North America
Recipes: Anti-itch creams

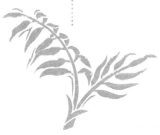

JUNIPER *(JUNIPERUS COMMUNIS)*
Parts Used: Berries, essential oil
Cosmetic Properties: Soothing, scent, antiseptic, cooling, refreshing
Grows: North America
Recipes: Bath and massage oils

KELP *(LAMINARIA DIGITATA)*
Parts Used: Seaweed flakes and powder
Cosmetic Properties: Emollient, rich in vitamins and minerals
Grows: Northern Atlantic and Pacific coasts
Recipes: Thalassotherapy body wraps and baths, herbal face lift

LADY'S MANTLE (ALCHEMILLA VULGARIS)
Parts Used: Flowering top
Cosmetic Properties: Astringent
Grows: Northeastern United States
Recipes: Baths

LAVENDER (LAVANDULA SPP.)
Parts Used: Flowers, stems, leaves, essential oil
Cosmetic Properties: Aromatic, restorative
Grows: North America, Europe
Recipes: Bath products, body powders, facial steams, masks

LEMON (CITRUS LIMON)
Parts Used: Pulp, peel, juice
Cosmetic Properties: Aromatic, astringent, bleaching,
pH balancing
Grows: Florida, California
Recipes: Bath products, facial steam, hair rinses, bleach

LEMON BALM (MELISSA OFFICINALIS)
Parts Used: Leaves, essential oil
Cosmetic Properties: Cleansing, antiseptic, fragrant
Grows: Temperate zones
Recipes: Facial steams, Queen of Hungary Water

LINDEN (TILIA X EUROPAEA)
Parts Used: Leaves and flowers
Cosmetic Properties: Aromatic, antiseptic, cooling, relaxing
Grows: Central and northeastern United States
Recipes: Facial treatments

LOOFAH (LUFFA AEGYPTIACA)
Parts Used: Fibrous gourd skeleton
Cosmetic Properties: Stimulating, exfoliant
Grows: Cultivated in North America
Recipes: Body scrubs

LOVAGE (LEVISTICUM OFFICINALE)
Parts Used: Leaves and stems
Cosmetic Properties: Exodorizer, fragrant

Grows: Native to Europe; cultivated in temperate zones
Recipes: Tea, floral water

MARSHMALLOW *(ALTHAEA OFFICINALIS)*
Parts Used: Root, flowering top
Cosmetic Properties: Emollient, soothing
Grows: Wild in northeastern United States
Recipes: Facial masks, steams

MYRRH *(COMMIPHORA MYRRHA)*
Parts Used: Resin, resin powder
Cosmetic Properties: Astringent, fragrant
Grows: Tropical
Recipes: Mouthwash, tooth powder

NETTLE *(URTICA DIOICA)*
Parts Used: Leaves
Cosmetic Properties: Stimulating, vitamin and mineral rich, improves circulation
Grows: Wild in most of United States
Recipes: Hair rinses

ORRIS *(IRIS X GERMANICA, I. PALLIDA)*
Parts Used: Powdered root
Cosmetic Properties: Aromatic, fixative
Grows: Temperate zones
Recipes: Body and foot powders

PARSLEY *(PETROSELINUM CRISPUM)*
Parts Used: Leaves
Cosmetic Properties: Cleansing, soothing, healing
Grows: Annual
Recipes: Hair rinses, blackhead treatment, eczema and psoriasis treatments

PATCHOULI *(POGOSTEMON CABLIN, P. PATCHOULI)*
Parts Used: Essential oil, leaves
Cosmetic Properties: Skin rejuvenator, scent, deodorant
Grows: Tropical regions
Recipes: Deodorant

PEPPERMINT *(MENTHA X PIPERITA)*

Parts Used: Leaves, essential oil
Cosmetic Properties: Stimulating, fragrant, deodorant
Grows: Temperate North America
Recipes: Facial masks and steams, body powder, mouthwash

PINE *(PINUS STROBUS)*

Parts Used: Needles, sap, essential oil
Cosmetic Properties: Stimulating, antiseptic, rich in vitamin C
Grows: Eastern North America
Recipes: Bath herbs, infused oils

POPPY *(ESCHSCHOLZIA CALIFORNICA, PAPAVER RHOEAS)*

Parts Used: Flower petals and seeds
Cosmetic Properties: Exfoliant, analgesic
Grows: Temperate zones
Recipes: Facial and body scrubs

QUASSIA *(PICRASMA EXCELSA)*

Parts Used: Bark
Cosmetic Properties: Cleansing, exfoliant
Grows: Jamaica
Recipes: Hair treatments

QUINCE *(CYDONIA OBLONGA)*

Parts Used: Seeds, flowers
Cosmetic Properties: Emollient
Grows: Temperate North America
Recipes: Lotions, creams

RASPBERRY *(RUBUS IDAEUS)*

Parts Used: Leaves, berries
Cosmetic Properties: Stimulating, astringent
Grows: Eastern North America
Recipes: Hair rinses, facial masks, steams, bath herb

RED CLOVER (TRIFOLIUM PRATENSE)
Parts Used: Blossoms, flowering tops, flower essence
Cosmetic Properties: Stimulating, promotes healing
Grows: Wild in temperate North America
Recipes: Scalp treatment

ROSE (ROSA SPP.)
Parts Used: Petals, essential oil, hips
Cosmetic Properties: Emollient, softening, restorative, fragrant
Grows: Temperate regions
Recipes: Facial masks, steams, body wraps

ROSEMARY (ROSMARINUS OFFICINALIS)
Parts Used: Needles, essential oil
Cosmetic Properties: Stimulating, astringent, conditioning
Grows: Wild in California and mild regions; indoors in harsher climates
Recipes: Facial masks, steams, bath herb

SAGE (SALVIA OFFICINALIS)
Parts Used: Leaves, flowers
Cosmetic Properties: Astringent
Grows: Temperate North America
Recipes: After-bath splash

SANDALWOOD (SANTALUM ALBUM)
Parts Used: Inner bark, essential oil
Cosmetic Properties: Disinfectant, antiseptic, fragrant
Grows: Tropical areas
Recipes: Bath herb

SPEARMINT (MENTHA SPICATA)
Parts Used: Leaves, essential oil
Cosmetic Properties: Stimulating, fragrant, deodorant
Grows: Temperate North America
Recipes: Facial masks and steams, mouthwash

ST.-JOHN'S-WORT *(HYPERICUM PERFORATUM)*
Parts Used: Flowering tops
Cosmetic Properties: Restorative, sun protection
Grows: Northern North America
Recipes: Sunscreen, scalp oil

STEVIA *(STEVIA REBAUDIANA)*
Parts Used: Dried leaves and twigs
Cosmetic Properties: Sweetener
Grows: Paraguay, Peru, Columbia, Mexico
Recipes: Skin tea

THUJA *(THUJA OCCIDENTALIS)*
Parts Used: Leaves, tops
Cosmetic Properties: Antifungal
Grows: United States and Europe
Recipes: Nail creams, footbaths, warts

THYME *(THYMUS VULGARIS)*
Parts Used: Flowers, leaves, essential oil
Cosmetic Properties: Aromatic, antiseptic, stimulant, disinfectant
Grows: Cultivated and wild in North America
Recipes: Deodorant, mouthwash, bath herb

VETIVERT *(VETIVERIA ZIZANIOIDES)*
Parts Used: Root, essential oil
Cosmetic Properties: Emollient, soothing, fragrant
Grows: Tropical areas
Recipes: Bath herb

VIOLET *(VIOLA ODORATA)*
Parts Used: Flowers, leaves
Cosmetic Properties: Emollient, slightly astringent
Grows: Naturalized in North America
Recipes: Eye cream

WINTERGREEN *(GAULTHERIA PROCUMBENS, PYROLA SPP.)*

Parts Used: Leaves, essential oil
Cosmetic Properties: Astringent, aromatic
Grows: Wild in the northeastern United States
Recipes: Tooth powder, lotions, creams

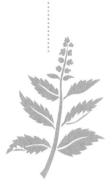

WITCH HAZEL *(HAMAMELIS VIRGINIANA)*

Parts Used: Inner bark, leaves
Cosmetic Properties: Styptic, cleansing, astringent
Grows: Nova Scotia to Georgia
Recipes: Footbaths, aftershave, skin toner

YARROW *(ACHILLEA MILLEFOLIUM)*

Parts Used: Flowers, flowering top
Cosmetic Properties: Astringent, cleansing, stimulating
Grows: Temperate regions
Recipes: Bath herb, shampoo, mouthwash

YELLOW DOCK *(RUMEX CRISPUS)*

Parts Used: Root
Cosmetic Properties: Alterative
Grows: Wild in temperate zones
Recipes: Skin tea

YLANG-YLANG *(CANANGA ODORATA)*

Parts Used: Flowers and essential oil
Cosmetic Properties: Aromatic
Grows: Madagascar
Recipes: Hair treatment, scent

YUCCA *(YUCCA SPP.)*

Parts Used: Roots
Cosmetic Properties: Emollient, cleansing
Grows: Southwestern United States
Recipes: Hair care

OVERVIEW OF FRUITS, NUTS, AND VEGETABLES

ALMOND *(PRUNUS DULCIS)*
Parts Used: Raw ground nuts, meal
Cosmetic Properties: Emollient, exfoliant
Grows: California
Where to Find: Health food stores, mail order
Recipes: Facial scrubs, masks

APPLE *(MALUS SYLVESTRIS)*
Parts Used: Organic pulp, juice
Cosmetic Properties: Slightly acidic, soothing especially for sensitive and fair skin
Grows: Northeast and northwestern United States
Where to Find: Health food stores, organic producers
Recipes: Masks, hand creams, scrubs, pomades

APRICOT *(PRUNUS ARMENIACA)*
Parts Used: Organic pulp, juice
Cosmetic Properties: Good for oily and sallow skin
Grows: Abundantly in California
Where to Find: Health food stores, organic producers
Recipes: Scrubs, masks

ARTICHOKE *(CYNARA SCOLYMUS)*
Parts Used: Organic leaves, heart, infusion
Cosmetic Properties: Rinse for dandruff
Grows: Cultivated in temperate zones
Where to Find: Health food stores, organic producers
Recipes: Hair rinse

ASPARAGUS *(ASPARAGUS OFFICINALIS)*
Parts Used: Spear, infusion
Cosmetic Properties: Stimulating, dries up pimples and sores
Grows: Temperate zones
Where to Find: Health food stores, organic producers
Recipes: Facial water and masques

AVOCADO *(PERSEA AMERICANA)*
Parts Used: Pulp, ground pit
Cosmetic Properties: Nourishing and conditioning for skin and hair; pit is nourishing, conditioning, exfoliant
Grows: California
Where to Find: Health food stores, organic producers
Recipes: Facial masks, hair masks

BANANA *(MUSA SPP.)*
Parts Used: Mashed pulp, skin
Cosmetic Properties: Nourishing, emollient
Grows: Tropical zones
Where to Find: Health food stores, organic producers
Recipes: Facial, body, and hair masks

BEET *(BETA VULGARIS)*
Parts Used: Pulp, juice
Cosmetic Properties: Tonic, colorant
Grows: Temperate zones
Where to Find: Health food stores, organic producers
Recipes: Facial masks, rouge, lipstick

BLACKBERRY *(RUBUS FRUTICOSUS)*
Parts Used: Leaves, berries
Cosmetic Properties: Astringent, cleansing, colorant
Grows: Northeastern United States
Where to Find: Health food stores, organic producers, wildcraft
Recipes: Facials, masks, lotions, steams

CARROT *(DAUCUS CAROTA)*
Parts Used: Mashed whole carrot
Cosmetic Properties: Antiseptic, effective on sores and skin ulcers
Grows: Temperate zones
Where to Find: Health food stores, organic producers
Recipes: Masks

CASHEW (ANACARDIUM OCCIDENTALE)
Parts Used: Ground meal
Cosmetic Properties: Exfoliant, emollient
Grows: Tropical areas
Where to Find: Health food stores, organic producers
Recipes: Facial scrubs, foot scrubs

CELERY (APIUM GRAVEOLENS)
Parts Used: Tops, infusion
Cosmetic Properties: Tonic, toning
Grows: Temperate zones
Where to Find: Health food stores, organic producers
Recipes: Creams, lotions, facial steams

CORN (ZEA MAYS)
Parts Used: Ground cornmeal, cornstarch
Cosmetic Properties: Exfoliant, emollient
Grows: Temperate zones
Where to Find: Health food stores, organic producers
Recipes: Masks, facial packs, body and foot powder

CUCUMBER (CUCUMIS SATIVUS)
Parts Used: Strained pulp, juice, slices
Cosmetic Properties: Bleaching, soothing, cooling, anti-itch, antiwrinkle
Grows: Temperate zones
Where to Find: Health food stores, organic producers
Recipes: Creams, lotions, masks

FIGS (FICUS CARICA)
Parts Used: Mashed pulp, juice
Cosmetic Properties: Emollient
Grows: Native to the Mediterranean region
Where to Find: Health food stores, organic producers
Recipes: Facial masks

GARLIC (ALLIUM SATIVUM)
Parts Used: Cloves

Cosmetic Properties: Stimulant, carminative, antiseptic, diaphoretic
Grows: Temperate zones
Where to Find: Health food stores, organic producers
Recipes: Hair rinse, facial wash

GRAPE (VITIS VINIFERA)
Parts Used: Mashed fruit, leaves, juice
Cosmetic Properties: Cooling, demulcent
Grows: Temperate zones
Where to Find: Health food stores, organic producers
Recipes: Masks, facial wash

LEMON (CITRUS LIMON)
Parts Used: Juice, pulp, zest
Cosmetic Properties: Astringent, bleaching, scent, disinfectant, antidandruff, acidic
Grows: California, Florida
Where to Find: Health food stores, organic producers
Recipes: Baths, facial steams, scrubs, masks

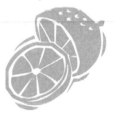

MELON (CUCUMIS MELO) CASABA, HONEYDEW, CANTALOUPE
Parts Used: Mashed pulp, juice
Cosmetic Properties: Emollient, especially for dry skin
Grows: North America
Where to Find: Health food stores, organic producers
Recipes: Facial masks, scrubs

ORANGE (CITRUS SINENSIS)
Parts Used: Blossoms, pulp, juice, zest
Cosmetic Properties: Emollient, antiseptic, aromatic, hydrating, astringent
Grows: California, Florida
Where to Find: Health food stores, organic producers
Recipes: Facial masks, shampoos, creams, hair rinses

PAPAYA *(CARICA PAPAYA)*
Parts Used: Strained pulp, leaves
Cosmetic Properties: Exfoliant, protein digesting
Grows: Tropical areas
Where to Find: Health food stores, organic producers
Recipes: Facial masks, cuticle cream

PEACH *(PRUNUS PERSICA)*
Parts Used: Pulp, juice
Cosmetic Properties: Enriching, moisturizing, toning
Grows: Southeastern United States
Where to Find: Health food stores, organic producers
Recipes: Facial masks, washes

PEANUT *(ARACHIS HYPOGAEA)*
Parts Used: Ground meal
Cosmetic Properties: Exfoliant, emollient
Grows: Southeastern United States
Where to Find: Health food stores, organic producers
Recipes: Facial masks

PEAR *(PYRUS COMMUNIS)*
Parts Used: Mashed pulp, juice
Cosmetic Properties: Soothing, cooling
Grows: Temperate zones
Where to Find: Health food stores, organic producers
Recipes: Facial masks

PINEAPPLE *(ANANAS COMOSUS)*
Parts Used: Pulp, juice
Cosmetic Properties: Astringent, bleaching
Grows: Hawaii
Where to Find: Health food stores, organic producers
Recipes: Facial scrub

PUMPKIN *(CUCURBITA PEPO)*
Parts Used: Mashed pulp
Cosmetic Properties: Emollient
Grows: Temperate zones
Recipes: Body treatments

RASPBERRY *(RUBUS IDAEUS)*
Parts Used: Leaves, fruit
Cosmetic Properties: Astringent
Grows: Temperate zones
Where to Find: Health food stores, organic producers
Recipes: Hair rinses, gargle

RHUBARB *(RHEUM RHABARBARUM)*
Parts Used: Roots and stalks
Cosmetic Properties: Astringent, brings out hair highlights
Grows: Cultivated in temperate zones
Recipes: Hair rinses

STRAWBERRY *(FRAGARIA VESCA)*
Parts Used: Leaves, fruit
Cosmetic Properties: Soothing, astringent
Grows: Wild and cultivated
Recipes: Bath herb, teeth whitening, facial masks

SUNFLOWER *(HELIANTHUS ANNUUS)*
Parts Used: Ground raw seeds
Cosmetic Properties: Exfoliant, emollient
Grows: Temperate zones
Where to Find: Health food stores, organic producers
Recipes: Facial masks

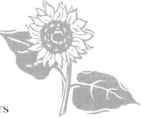

TOMATO *(LYCOPERSICON LYCOPERSICUM)*
Parts Used: Juice, pulp
Cosmetic Properties: Astringent
Grows: Cultivated
Recipes: Facial masks

WATERMELON *(CITRULLUS LANATUS)*
Parts Used: Mashed pulp, juice
Cosmetic Properties: Emollient, especially for oily skin
Grows: Cultivated
Recipes: Facial masks, scrubs

OVERVIEW OF GRAINS AND BEANS

ADZUKI BEANS *(VIGNA ANGULARIS)*
Parts Used: Ground beans
Cosmetic Properties: Exfoliant
Where to Find: Health food stores
Recipes: Oriental cleansing grains

BARLEY *(HORDEUM VULGARE)*
Parts Used: Ground barley
Cosmetic Properties: Exfoliant
Where to Find: Grocery and health food stores
Recipes: Facial scrubs

CHICK PEAS *(CICER ARIETINUM)*
Parts Used: Dried ground chick peas
Cosmetic Properties: Exfoliant, emollient
Where to Find: Grocery and health food stores
Recipes: Body and facial scrubs

FLOUR
Cosmetic Properties: Moisturizing
Where to Find: Grocery and health food stores
Recipes: Hair treatments

OATS *(AVENA SATIVA)*
Parts Used: Ground dry oatmeal or bran
Cosmetic Properties: Exfoliant, emollient
Where to Find: Grocery and health food stores;
growing wild
Recipes: Facial and body scrubs

PEAS *(PISUM SATIVUM)*
Parts Used: Cooked and mashed pea
Cosmetic Properties: Emollient
Where to Find: Grocery and health food stores
Recipes: Facial masks, washes

RICE *(ORYZA SATIVA)*
Parts Used: Ground rice
Cosmetic Properties: Exfoliant, emollient
Where to Find: Grocery and health food stores
Recipes: Facial and body masks, scrubs

OVERVIEW OF OILS AND BUTTERS

ALMOND OIL *(PRUNUS DULCIS)*
Parts Used: Oil pressed from almonds
Cosmetic Properties: Emollient, light in color, fragrant
Where to Find: Specialty gourmet and health food stores, mail order
Recipes: Moisturizers, body care

APRICOT KERNEL OIL OR PERSIC OIL *(PRUNUS ARMENIACA)*
Parts Used: Oil pressed from apricot kernel
Cosmetic Properties: Emollient, light in color, fragrant
Where to Find: Specialty gourmet and health food stores, mail order
Recipes: Moisturizers, massage oil, body care

AVOCADO OIL *(PERSEA AMERICANA)*
Parts Used: Oil from flesh
Cosmetic Properties: Emollient, pale green, absorbs UV radiation, antioxidant, moisturizing
Where to Find: Specialty gourmet and health food stores, mail order
Recipes: Moisturizers, hair care, body care

BORAGE OIL *(BORAGO OFFICINALIS)*
Parts Used: Oil pressed from plant
Cosmetic Properties: Emollient, demulcent, diuretic, diaphoretic
Where to Find: Specialty gourmet and health food stores, mail order
Recipes: Nail oil, face and body moisturizers

CANOLA OIL

Parts Used: Oil pressed from the bean
Cosmetic Properties: Emollient, light in color, fragrant
Where to Find: Supermarkets, health food stores,
mail order
Recipes: Face and body moisturizers

CASTOR BEAN OIL *(RICINUS COMMUNIS)*

Parts Used: Oil pressed from the bean
Cosmetic Properties: Thickener, emollient
Where to Find: Drug and health food stores, mail order
Recipes: Hair and nail care

COCOA BUTTER *(THEOBROMA CACAO)*

Parts Used: Fatty wax
Cosmetic Properties: Emolliant, skin softener, solid at
room temperature
Where to Find: Drug and health food stores, mail order
Recipes: Moisturizers, body care

COCONUT OIL *(COCS NUCIFERA)*

Parts Used: Oil
Cosmetic Properties: Emollient, conditioning, protecting
Where to Find: Specialty gourmet and health food stores,
mail order
Recipes: Face moisturizer, creamy lotions

CORN OIL *(ZEA MAYS)*

Parts Used: Oil; use only organic corn — other types may be
sprayed with pesticides and insecticides
Cosmetic Properties: Emollient
Where to Find: Health food stores, mail order
Recipes: Nail oil

GRAPESEED OIL *(VITIS VINIFERA)*

Parts Used: Oil pressed from grapeseed
Cosmetic Properties: Emollient, nonallergenic, light green
hue, least greasy oil

Where to Find: Specialty gourmet and health food stores, mail order
Recipes: Massage, body care

JOJOBA BEAN OIL *(SIMMONDSIA CHINENSIS)*
Parts Used: Oil extracted from shrub pod
Cosmetic Properties: Emollient, similar to natural human oil secretions, antioxidant
Grows: Southern California, Arizona, New Mexico, Mexico
Where to Find: Specialty gourmet and health food stores, mail order; in area where it grows, you can find it locally
Recipes: Body and hair care, moisturizer

OLIVE OIL *(OLEA EUROPAEA)*
Parts Used: Cold pressed virgin oil
Cosmetic Properties: Emollient, restorative, moderately fragrant, yellow-green hue
Where to Find: Specialty gourmet and health food stores, mail order
Recipes: Body and hair care

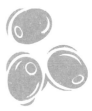

PUMPKIN SEED OIL *(CUCURBITA PEPO)*
Parts Used: Oil extracted from the seed
Cosmetic Properties: Emollient
Where to Find: Specialty gourmet and health food stores, mail order
Recipes: Body care

SAFFLOWER OIL *(CARTHAMUS TINCTORIUS)*
Parts Used: Oil
Cosmetic Properties: Emollient
Where to Find: Grocery, specialty gourmet, and health food stores; mail order
Recipes: Body care

SESAME OIL *(SESAMUM INDICUM)*

Parts Used: Oil extracted from sesame seeds, not the toasted or cooking oil but the light skin-care oil
Cosmetic Properties: Emollient, absorbs UV radiation, sunscreen
Where to Find: Health food stores, mail order
Recipes: Sunscreen products, moisturizer

SHEA BUTTER OR AFRICAN KARITE BUTTER *(BOTYROSPERMUM PARKII)*

Parts Used: Pressed from the pits of the fruit
Cosmetic Properties: Emollient
Where to Find: Specialty gourmet and health food stores, mail order
Recipes: Hair treatments

SUNFLOWER OIL *(HELIANTHUS ANNUUS)*

Parts Used: Oil extracted from sunflower seeds
Cosmetic Properties: Emollient
Where to Find: Specialty gourmet and health food stores, mail order
Recipes: Nail oil

VITAMIN E OIL

Parts Used: Only 100 percent natural d-alpha tocopherol; other forms are synthetic.
Cosmetic Properties: Preservative, prevents scarring, slows aging
Where to Find: Specialty gourmet and health food stores, mail order
Recipes: Lip balms, moisturizing creams, lotions

WHEAT GERM OIL *(TRITICUM AESTIVUM)*

Parts Used: Oil extracted from wheat germ
Cosmetic Properties: Emollient, rich in vitamin E, antioxidant
Where to Find: Specialty gourmet and health food stores, mail order
Recipes: Nail oil

Refer to the bibliography for references.

OVERVIEW OF SALTS AND
MISCELLANEOUS INGREDIENTS

APPLE CIDER VINEGAR
Parts Used: Diluted vinegar
Cosmetic Properties: Astringent, anti-itch, slightly acid pH similar to that of skin
Where to Find: Grocery and health food stores
Recipes: Baths, facial toner

BAKING SODA (SODIUM BICARBONATE)
Parts Used: Crystalline powder
Cosmetic Properties: Soothing, water softening, effervescent, deodorizing, stimulating; draws oils and impurities from the skin
Where to Find: Grocery store
Recipes: Bath crystals, body powders, tooth powders

BEESWAX
Parts Used: Wax refined or unrefined
Cosmetic Properties: Thickener
Source: Honeycomb
Where to Find: Apiary, craft store, herbal supply store
Recipes: Moisturizers

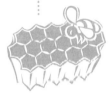

BENZOIN GUM
Parts Used: Resin from trees of the genus *Styrax*
Cosmetic Properties: Antiseptic, preservative
Grows: Tropical Asia
Where to Find: Health food stores, mail order
Recipes: Moisturizers, lotions

BORAX (SODIUM TETRABORATE), DESERT SALT
Parts Used: Crystalline powder
Cosmetic Properties: Antiseptic, water softening, deodorizing
Source: Natural desert mineral salts
Where to Find: Laundry section of grocery store
Recipes: Bath crystals

CASTILE SOAP

Parts Used: Commercial or homemade liquid or bars
Cosmetic Properties: Gentle cleanser
Source: Natural olive oil base
Where to Find: Health food stores, mail order
Recipes: Shampoos, bubble baths

CLAY

Parts Used: Dried powder
Types: *Bentonite* — gentle gray, actually not clay but similar; *French White* — gentle white; *Kaolin* — gentle white; *Green* — stronger green; *Red* — stronger red; *Black* — medium black from the Dead Sea, rich in minerals
Cosmetic Properties: Stimulating, draws oils and impurities from the skin
Source: Volcanic product
Recipes: Facial scrubs, masks, body powders

CREAM OF TARTAR

Parts Used: Powder
Cosmetic Properties: Stabilizer, effervescent
Source: By-product of wine fermentation
Where to Find: Grocery store
Recipes: Body wraps

EPSOM SALTS (MAGNESIUM SULFATE)

Parts Used: Crystalline salts
Cosmetic Properties: Relieves aches and pains, stimulating, draws oils and impurities from the skin
Source: Synthetic preparation
Where to Find: Grocery, drug, and discount department stores
Recipes: Bath crystals, footbaths

FLORAL WATERS: ROSE, LAVENDER, ORANGE BLOSSOM

Parts Used: Blossoms
Cosmetic Properties: Hydrating, emollient
Where to Find: Gourmet shops, herb catalogs, or make it yourself (see pages 99–100)
Recipes: Body and face moisturizers, hand creams

FOLIC ACID
Parts Used: Powder
Cosmetic Properties: Sunscreen
Source: B vitamin
Where to Find: Pharmacy
Recipes: Sunscreen, face moisturizer

GELATIN, UNFLAVORED
Parts Used: Powder
Cosmetic Properties: Emollient, nourisher
Source: Skin, bones, and connective tissue of animals
Recipes: Peel-off mask, nail treatments

GLYCERIN
Parts Used: Syrupy liquid
Cosmetic Properties: Emollient, humectant, sweetener, preservative
Source: Animal and vegetable fats
Recipes: Facial masks

MAYONNAISE
Parts Used: Commercial or homemade product made from oil, eggs, and vinegar or lemon juice
Cosmetic Properties: Emollient, restores natural pH
Recipes: Hair packs, facial masks

MILK AND CREAM
Parts Used: Powdered, whole, and skim milk; heavy cream
Cosmetic Properties: Emollient
Source: Usually cow, but goat is equally good
Recipes: Baths, facials

PABA POWDER
Parts Used: Powder
Cosmetic Properties: Sunscreen
Source: B vitamin
Where to Find: Pharmacy
Recipes: Sunscreen

PARAFFIN WAX

Parts Used: Melted wax
Cosmetic Properties: Moisturizing
Where to Find: Grocery store
Recipes: Hand and foot treatments

YOGURT (PLAIN)

Parts Used: Any
Cosmetic Properties: Emollient, mildly astringent
Grows: By fermenting milk with bacteria
Recipes: Facial and body scrubs, masks

ZINC OXIDE PASTE

Parts Used: White paste
Cosmetic Properties: Sunblock
Where to Find: Pharmacy
Recipes: Sunblock

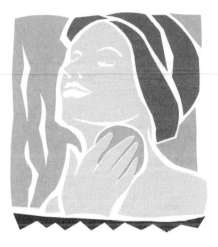

Getting Set Up to Make and Enjoy Your Spa Treatments

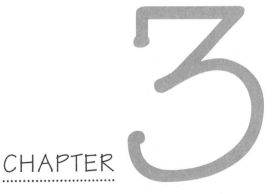

CHAPTER 3

Making your own body-care products is easy, fun, nurturing, and liberating. I am not an enthusiastic cook; the day-to-day aspects of cooking do not excite me. Nourishment is important to me, though, so I cook. Creating herbal products, however, is another story. I have an enormous amount of fun, experience independence, and feel great freedom and success in creating these products. Please don't feel you have to be a great cook. Trust me, I have had many more food flops than I have herbal cosmetics flops. Read this chapter carefully before you dive into the specific recipes in subsequent chapters, so you can establish your work area, have the right equipment on hand, and get your home spa set up for maximum enjoyment.

ASSEMBLING THE EQUIPMENT

To get started making your own herbal body-care products you need look no further than your kitchen for the basic equipment; no special equipment or great cooking skills are required to create the recipes in this book. All you'll need are some common kitchen appliances and equipment and a desire to create.

It is best to reserve the equipment you use for making herbal products solely for this purpose, especially any plastic tools such as spatulas and blenders; glass equipment is easier to clean and sterilize. Some of the essential oils used in many of the recipes may leave a residue that is better left out of your meals. The equipment doesn't have to be new when you start, but once you've used it for this purpose, I don't recommend using it for food preparation. Following are the pieces of equipment you will need.

BLENDER

Used for making moisturizing creams and lotions. Also may be used to grind herbs and grains loosely or to a fine powder. A glass blender is far easier to clean than is the plastic variety.

CUTTING BOARD

It is nice to have several boards of different sizes that can be moved around as needed. I prefer those made of wood, which can be replaced when they become too worn. If you use your cutting

Equipment for making herbal products can be found in most well-equipped kitchens.

board for both meat and herbal products, use plastic cutting boards, which are easier to sanitize and maintain than wood.

DOUBLE BOILER

Produces gentle, even heat, which is especially helpful in making infused herbal oil products such as massage oils, lip balms, eye creams, and moisturizers. It is important that your double boiler be either stainless steel, enamel, or glass. Do not use aluminum, copper, Teflon, or cast iron; these will affect the finished product.

EYEDROPPERS OR PIPETTES

Glass eyedroppers or pipettes are useful for measuring essential oils and resins. These can be purchased through herbal suppliers and bottle and container suppliers.

FUNNELS

You can purchase a set of three sizes of funnels, which will come in handy for filling bottles and containers. I have had a hard time finding widemouthed funnels, but they are easy to make using recycled gallon or half-gallon plastic containers (the kind milk comes in). Simply cut the plastic, maintaining the handle and spout opening. You can also create a scoop/funnel this way.

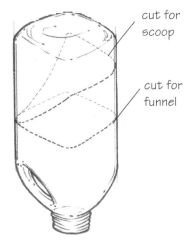

cut for scoop

cut for funnel

GLASS BOWLS

Glass bowls are especially nice to use — and easy to clean — but stainless-steel bowls will also work. You'll need a variety of bowls, from custard size to large mixing bowls.

GLOVES

Dishwashing gloves are okay; however, the closer-fitting latex type allows for fine movements and better dexterity.

GRATER

Useful in grating soap and vegetables. I prefer a plastic grater to the metal one, but either will work. Many books suggest grating beeswax. I usually end up grating my fingers when I attempt this. Instead, I cut the beeswax into small pieces using a paring knife.

MEASURING CUPS AND SPOONS

Helpful in keeping ingredients in proportion to each other. In some recipes, exact measurements can ensure success.

MORTAR AND PESTLE

Great for crushing dried herbs, seeds, flowers, and bark, as well as fresh fruit and vegetable pulps. I recommend the marble variety, although I also have an excellent wooden set.

PARING KNIVES

Great for cutting and chopping herbs, flowers, and fruits; use to sliver beeswax.

SAUCEPANS

Stainless-steel or enamel pans are best. Large spaghetti pots are good for making floral and aromatic waters; smaller pans are also useful.

SPATULA

You can't have too many spatulas. Very useful for scooping and filling containers.

SPICE MILL OR COFFEE GRINDER

A blender will work, but a spice mill is preferable for grinding oatmeal, almonds, lavender,
roses, and any number of other herbs, grains,
and seeds. Enjoy the fragrance of the powdered flowers and aromatic herbs. Note: To
clean the inner workings of the mill, do not
wash or immerse it; simply wipe it clean with
a dry cloth. Washing or exposing to water will
ruin the engine and you'll soon be traveling to
the store for a new one. Be aware that if you
use the same grinder for coffee beans, your
herbal products will contain a hint of coffee
and your coffee a hint of herbs.

WARNING

Do not use pans and other
equipment with copper, aluminum, Teflon, or cast-iron
finishes. These materials
react with the ingredients
in your recipe and will ad-
versely affect the quality of
the finished product.

STIRRING RODS

Chopsticks, wood or plastic, work well for dispersing scents in
oil, but glass chemistry stirring rods are even better and are easier to clean. This is where it pays to have a brother who works
in a lab! (Thanks, Larry.) If you're not so lucky, look for labora-
tory suppliers in the Yellow Pages. Be sure to use new rods that
have never been used in toxic chemicals!

STRAINERS

Various meshes and sizes come in very handy, especially in
making herbal infusions and grinding nuts. The Vermont Country Store (see resource list) carries a nice set of three at about
half the price you'll pay at gourmet cooking shops.

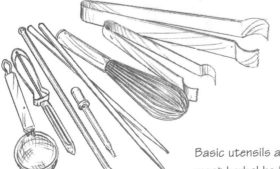

Basic utensils are sufficient for
most herbal body-care recipes.

TONGS

The long barbecue type are best for use in body wraps, but the shorter variety will also help protect your hands from hot water.

VEGETABLE PEELER OR ZESTER

Great for removing the zest from citrus fruits and vegetables.

WIRE WHISK

Essential for mixing bath crystals and facial and body scrubs. Helps to distribute the scent throughout these products; besides, it's fun to use.

SELECTING STORAGE CONTAINERS

Bottles and containers can get quite pricey, especially if you make herbal products to give as gifts or to sell. I am always on the lookout for pretty containers. Occasionally, you may find bottles at discount stores, gourmet shops, and gift and specialty stores. I purchase most of my bottles from a local wholesaler, but this requires buying by the case. There are several retail mail-order suppliers that sell containers in smaller quantities (see resource list).

It is helpful to know the common names used to refer to various bottle shapes and styles. Following are descriptions of the ones I use most often.

RECYCLING BOTTLES AND CONTAINERS

When creating products for yourself, recycled containers can be a godsend. Some of my most beautiful containers are finds from flea markets and tag sales. Before you package what you've made, however, be sure to sterilize the container (see page 52). If you are inspired to start your own product line to sell, the FDA requires that you use new containers only.

Glass Containers

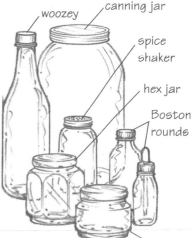

woozey
canning jar
spice shaker
hex jar
Boston rounds
cream jar

Clear glass containers are readily available, but glass in amber and in blue is becoming more popular. These colored glasses better protect products containing oils and dried herbs from light.

CREAM JARS

These pretty jars with wide mouths are excellent for creams and salves.

SPICE SHAKERS

These shakers are usually 2 inches high and are perfect for sprinkling out dried herbs that you might use in small quantities. These containers can be used to dispense your powder preparations because of the shaker tops.

WOOZEYS

These narrow-necked jars are designed for herbal vinegars and wines and come in different sizes. The most common are 5-ounce, 10-ounce, and 12-ounce versions. They can be used for culinary vinegars, bath vinegars, and bath oils.

HEX JARS

These six-sided, widemouthed jars are used by beekeepers for storing honey because of their resemblance to the honeycomb. They are very pretty and useful for creams and moisturizers, although I find the lids to be unreliable for travel.

STORAGE OR CANNING JARS

These jars are usually available in pint, quart, half-gallon, and gallon sizes. I use them to store dried herbs.

BOSTON ROUNDS

These glass jars are available in clear, amber, and cobalt blue. They come in many sizes, from ½ ounce to 16 ounces with either a glass dropper or simply a cap. The colored glass protects products from bright light.

Plastic Containers

CREAM JARS

These opaque, white, widemouthed jars are great for lip balms, salves, and moisture creams. They are especially convenient for travel.

LOTION BOTTLES

Translucent, squeezable, flip-top bottles are perfect for creamy lotions and massage oils.

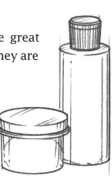

Other Containers

TINS

Shallow, widemouthed, decorative tins containing a label on the cover are great for salves and lip balms.

POWDER CYLINDERS

These white, lined, cardboard cylinders are excellent containers for herbal body powders and bath crystals. The white cardboard is easy to decorate with stickers or labels.

PRESS-AND-BREW TEA BAGS

These ready-to-make tea bags can be used to create your own tea blends or eye bags. Just place 1 to 2 teaspoons of the herbs in the bag and iron the closure. These are available in several different sizes from herbal suppliers. (See the resources list at the back of the book.)

MUSLIN BAGS

Also available in a variety of sizes, these drawstring bags are useful for making herbal tea (1 cup to 1 gallon) and herbal bath bags.

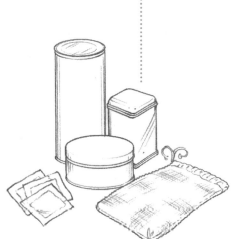

Decorating Containers

This book is full of gift ideas. Since so many of the products you can make are packaged in jars, bottles, tins, or clear plastic bags, stickers are a great way to personalize and decorate your wares. There are many unusual stickers available today, both humorous and beautiful; the search for just the right one for a particular friend can be rewarding and fun.

Find a sticker that illustrates the use for or an ingredient in your product — a hand, a basket of herbs, a bee — or symbolizes something special about your friend — a favorite animal or hobby, for example. Stickers can be found in so many different places: Discount department stores, drugstores, craft stores, stationery stores, and gift shops often carry a variety. Or try your hand at creating your own from blank white labels (available in many different sizes at a stationery store). Children especially like to decorate their own stickers.

Ribbons are an elegant addition to your packaging. Start saving a variety of ribbons and bows. Be sure to recycle any ribbons you receive on gifts. Let your friends know you're collecting, and you may be surprised at the assortment you get from them. If you want to create a down-to-earth look, raffia is just the thing for you. Ribbons and stickers often work well together for that finishing touch.

USING RECYCLED CONTAINERS

Avoid reusing containers that previously held medicine, film, poison, household cleaners, spoiled food, compost, or fertilizer. Use common sense to decide whether a container is safe to reuse.

Always sterilize any container that has been previously used to ensure the purity of your finished product. If you plan to sell your products, the FDA requires that you use new containers only. Following are the sterilization standards set up by the U.S. Occupational Health and Safety Administration (OSHA).

Sterilizing Glass Containers with Metal Lids

1. Wash the containers and lids thoroughly with soap and water, rinsing several times.
2. Combine ¼ cup bleach with 2 cups of hot water and submerge the clean containers and lids thoroughly in this solution.
3. Fill a large enamel or stainless-steel pot with water.
4. Submerse the bottles and lids, making sure there are no air bubbles left in the bottles.
5. Cover the pot and bring to a rolling boil.
6. Boil for 20 minutes; let cool.
7. Remove bottles and lids from water and allow to air-dry on a sterile towel.

Plastic Containers

Unfortunately, plastic containers are harder to sterilize because the boiling process may melt them. I recommend washing thoroughly and rinsing in the bleach formula; a good dishwashing cycle can also kill many harmful substances that cannot be seen. Use plastic containers to package products that are less prone to spoilage.

Watch for spoilage in your finished products and in the bulk ingredients. Make products in small batches to help reduce the potential for spoilage. If you are concerned about a product or if it smells off, throw it away: Better safe than sorry. If your herbs look old and withered or start to mold, offer them to the compost pile.

CREATING THE SPA EXPERIENCE AT HOME

Setting up a relaxing atmosphere is a major part of the spa experience. Many people feel they need to leave their home and the cares of the day behind. While it is important to create an ambience that feels different from your daily routine, with a little planning, a few props, and some clearly expressed boundaries with your family, you will be able to transform your home into a wonderful environment for relaxation. This can be accomplished quite easily and inexpensively, too.

Separate the Making from the Enjoying

It is so important to set things up in such a way that you get the full value of the experience while still doing it yourself. Whenever possible, separate the process of creating the products from the time set aside to use them. I really enjoy creating herbal products; the alchemist in me enjoys experimenting. Yet when it's time to use the products, out comes the inner princess. So by all means, enjoy the creation process and allow yourself to become fully absorbed in making your treatments. But remember also to allow yourself to switch gears, to let go of the "creator" role for a while, and luxuriate in the spa treatments when the time is right.

A SPECIAL MESSAGE FOR WOMEN

Women are drawn to spas because they provide one of their few opportunities to receive divinely feminine care. Too many women feel depleted because they themselves don't take the time to receive, because they are caught up in giving to others. This is especially true of mothers. If this rings true for you, accept this as a personal invitation to take in and receive the pleasures of nature.

If you find yourself resenting the people in your life, it may be because you never learned, first, how to give to yourself and, second, how to receive from them. Start taking more time for yourself and I promise that you will see a major change for the better in your relationships and even in your "luck." The busiest of women can and should find 5 to 10 minutes each day for personal pampering.

Open Yourself to the Experience

Part of the spa experience is being able to let go and take in the gifts that the herbs, flowers, and other ingredients have to offer you. My experience with plants is that their healing qualities and individuality are best expressed when you are open to receiving them. Being open to taking in the physical touch of a massage, rub, soak, or other treatment is also key to appreciating the spa experience.

Create the Mood

The key ingredients to create a setting that is relaxing are: lighting, music, color, aroma, comfortable surroundings and privacy, as well as gentle touch.

Lighting. Soft lighting sets a relaxing tone and is helpful in creating ambience. If you need brighter light to actually see what you're doing during the treatment, use a lamp or small light for the immediate area, and dim background lighting. Draping harsh lamps with a scarf can dim the light and set the mood for relaxation.

Candles are another great mood setter. Use care in placing the candles to avoid starting a fire. Candles are also a great way to diffuse fragrances you find calming. Aromatherapy candles abound, or you can simply add a few drops of your favorite scent to a candle. I like to use hurricane candles; they seem safer to me.

Music. Soft, relaxing music helps to set the mood. Some people prefer the peace of silence; for others, classical music is what really settles them down. I love silence, but that's not always possible to achieve, especially if you're doing the treatments when others are at home or if you live in a city or a noisy neighborhood. It is best to avoid music with lyrics, because singing along becomes an outward expression and we want to create the opposite. It pays to invest in a compact disc or two of music you find relaxing; try some of the New Age recordings. The music of Rob Whitesides-Woo or Kitaro takes me to a dreamy place. I also find most flute music soothing. Try several different selections to see what you find most relaxing.

Color. The color of your surroundings will also affect your mood. Recently, a local prison decided to paint the walls pink because this color discourages aggression and seems to foster relaxation. Color is used extensively in the fast-food and formal restaurant businesses: Reds, oranges, and golds stimulate appetite. Pink promotes relaxation. Chose a pink that is pleasing to you: Icy, hot, rosy, pastel, peach, coral, and salmon will all work. Hate pink? Choose a soft color that you love.

Drape the color around the area where you will be pampered. Throw a pink scarf over the lampshade and dim the light while bringing in the color at the same time. Or be really bold and decorate the room that you will be using for treatments in colors you find relaxing. The bathroom is a great place to create a sanctuary.

Aroma. Scents and aromas affect your mood. With the wide availability of pure essential oils and other aromatherapy products, you can easily create a scent atmosphere at home. Choose a fragrance that you find pleasing and calming. A scent may have a different effect on different people, depending on associations and life experiences, but lavender and chamomile are the fragrances most often chosen for relaxation. Bergamot, frankincense, neroli, patchouli, rose, sandalwood, and ylang-ylang are also relaxing. Patchouli, sandalwood, and frankincense are earthy; the others are more flowery. Visit a store that carries essential oils and use the tester to sample various scents. *Note:* Essential oils are highly concentrated; most should not be applied directly to the skin.

Comfortable surroundings. You know what this means for you: Maybe you like the casualness of country decor, or a more refined elegance, a dramatic setting, or funky, or art deco. Whatever your preference, create a setting that is both pleasing and offers privacy. Access to the bathroom is ideal for many of these treatments. If you have a large bathroom, you may want

> **MAKE YOUR SPA EXPERIENCE ENJOYABLE**
>
> Pamper yourself! Use
> - Large, fluffy towels
> - Tub pillow
> - Tub tray
> - Shower stool
> - Terry cloth robe
> - Turban
> - Slippers
> - Space heater
>
> or anything else that makes your spa special.

to make that your spa space. If you have a bedroom with an adjoining bath, you can use both rooms.

Privacy. Creating a space where you will not be disturbed is essential. Let your husband, housemates, or kids know that you are going to be off-limits for a while. Let them know how long you need. Put up a "Do not disturb" sign. Enlist your family's cooperation. Before you start your treatment, take the phone off the hook or put on the answering machine.

CREATING AROMATHERAPY

There are many ways to scent your home using essential oils. Check out your local health food store or perfume shop to learn about diffuser styles. Some diffusers require a tea light or votive candle, other are ceramic rings that can be placed over a lightbulb: The heat of the candle or bulb releases the scent. I prefer the candle over the electric choices.

For a lighter scent, small aromatic pottery works well. These small, bottle-shaped pieces of pottery are left partially unglazed. You simply uncork and add some essential oil. The essential oil seeps through the unglazed pottery and cork. This also works well for scenting your car.

The least expensive way to scent your home is to gently simmer herbs in a saucepan with water. Toss a handful of dried or two handfuls of fresh aromatic herbs in a saucepan full of boiling water, lower to simmer, and voilá! All the mints and aromatics work well with this technique, including lavender, rose, lovage, marjoram, sage, oregano, and thyme. Spices are also wonderfully effective, and you only need about a 1/4 cup. Cloves, cinnamon chips, aniseed and fennel seeds, bay leaf, and nutmeg can be used in combination or alone. If you are going to use the stove, you might want to create a floral water at the same time (see pages 99–100).

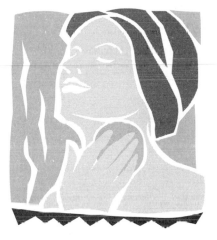

Herbs for the
Hair and Scalp

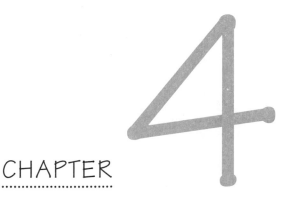

CHAPTER

Achieving great-looking hair is not difficult, nor does it need to be expensive. With a few common kitchen ingredients and some specialty oils, herbs, and flowers, you can create a variety of treatments that your hair will respond to quickly. The time you invest in creating these easy formulas will be rewarded with healthier, more radiant hair.

You can customize the basic herbal shampoo provided in this chapter to address your particular hair color, texture, and other individual needs. The herbal hair conditioner and rinse formulas should be applied after the shampoo to help keep the hair healthy from the roots to the ends. The scalp treatments here, including a flower essence massage, are designed to keep the scalp and new hair growth healthy. Some of them are formulated to address particular hair and scalp problems, such as controlling dandruff and encouraging hair growth. The final section of this chapter offers instructions for herbal hair coloring, a fun area to explore if you are an adventuresome do-it-yourselfer.

SHAMPOOING TECHNIQUE

For best results, try the following :

- Wet hair thoroughly and use a small amount of shampoo, a dollop about the size of a quarter.

- Put the shampoo on your hands. Rub them together to form a lather before applying to your hair.

- Use your fingertips, not your fingernails, to massage the shampoo into your scalp.

- Rinse hair thoroughly, then shampoo again.

- Rinse again thoroughly, using the coolest water possible for the shiniest hair.

- Pat hair dry; avoid rubbing.

- Gently comb hair, using a broad-tooth comb.

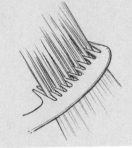

HERBAL SHAMPOOS

Shampoos are made to clean the scalp first and the hair second. I recommend customizing your shampoo recipe so that it offers optimal nourishment to your particular hair type and condition.

Selecting Customized Herbs for the Basic Shampoo Formula

Choose herbs for your shampoo that will enhance your hair color and texture, and that address any special needs you may have. You can mix and match herbs from the following lists to develop an individualized combination that is best for your hair.

INGREDIENTS FOR DIFFERENT HAIR TYPES

Dry	Normal	Oily	Ethnic
Comfrey root	Dandelion	Watercress	Comfrey
Avocado	Horse tail	Strawberry leaf	Nettle
Elder flowers	Clover	White willow bark	Cherry bark
Orange blossoms		Lemon grass	Olive oil

INGREDIENTS FOR SPECIAL CONDITIONS

Shine	Manage-ability	Softness	Dandruff	Growth
Egg	Yogurt	Cherry bark	White willow bark	St.-John's-wort
Raspberry	Cherry bark	Burdock root	Birch bark	Nettle
Nettle	Beer	Olive oil	Comfrey	Sage
Vinegar		Marjoram	Nettle	Basil
Quassia			Peppermint	Rosemary
			Vinegar	Onion juice

Blond	Brunet	Red	Darkest
Chamomile	Sage	Henna	Black malva
Calendula	Lavender	Calendula	Indigo
Lemon peel	Cinnamon chips	Red hibiscus	Lavender
Honey	Cloves	Cinnamon	Sage
Lemon juice	Rosemary	Beets	
Mullein flowers			

BASIC SHAMPOO FORMULA

2 tablespoons (30 ml) liquid castile soap

1 cup (250 ml) spring water

¼ cup (50 ml) fresh herbs (2 table-spoons [30 ml] dried)

1 teaspoon (5 ml) almond or apricot kernel oil

2 drops essential oil

Yield: Approximately 24 shampoos

To make:

1. Place herbs in a clean 10-ounce (284 g) glass jar with a lid.

2. Boil the spring water and pour over the herbs.

3. Cover and let steep for 10 to 20 minutes.

4. Strain the liquid from the herbs into a bowl.

5. Add the liquid castile soap and almond or apricot kernel oil and mix thoroughly.

6. Scent with essential oil and mix again.

7. Bottle in a plastic container with a spout or a clean recycled shampoo bottle.

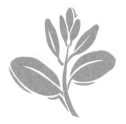

HERBAL HAIR CONDITIONERS

Herbal hair conditions help make hair more manageable and often impart a smoother and softer texture. They are especially good for those who cannnot live without hot rollers, curling irons, and blow dryers.

JOJOBA CONDITIONER

1 cup (250 ml) rose floral water (see recipe on page 100)

1 tablespoon (15 ml) jojoba oil

10 drops vitamin E oil

Yield: 1 treatment for long hair (cut recipe in half for short hair)

To make:

1. In the top of a double boiler, gently warm the rose water.

2. Once rose water is warm, add jojoba oil.

3. Pour the mixture in a blender and add the vitamin E. Blend at high speed for 2 minutes.

To use:

1. Wet hair with warm water.

2. Pour the conditioner onto your hair and scalp, massaging in thoroughly.

3. For damaged hair or extra conditioning, leave on for several minutes, perhaps while bathing.

4. Rinse thoroughly with warm water.

5. Shampoo lightly and rinse again with cool water.

MAYONNAISE HAIR PACK

A longtime favorite of my husband's grandmother Bessie, mayonnaise is a great conditioner for dry hair, and the vinegar helps the hair maintain its proper pH.

1 cup (250 ml) mayonnaise (make your own fresh or use a premade natural product)

Yield: 1 treatment

To use:

1. Wet hair with warm water.
2. Scoop mayonnaise into a small dish.
3. Dip your fingertips (not nails) into the bowl.
4. Gently massage the mayonnaise all over your scalp, working in a circular motion.
5. Massage the mayonnaise into the hair shaft and the ends.
6. Cover your hair with a plastic bag and allow the mayonnaise to stay on the scalp for at least ½ hour.
7. Shampoo as you normally would.
8. Repeat weekly, or as often as desired.

FLOURING

More the rage in Europe, especially France, than in North America, flouring is used for making the hair manageable and shiny. Most any flour will work, but I prefer white spelt and barley for added softness.

½ cup (125 ml) white spelt flour

½ cup (125 ml) barley flour

½ cup (125 ml) distilled water

½ cup (125 ml) rose or lavender floral water (see recipe on page 100)

1 tablespoon (15 ml) apple cider vinegar

1 plastic bag that can fit over the hair

Yield: 1 treatment for long hair

To make:

1. Sift the flours together in a large bowl.

2. Pour the distilled water, floral water, and vinegar over the flours.

To use:

1. Spoon the flour mixture onto your dry hair.

2. Smooth the paste all over the hair shaft. (This treatment is for the hair. It is not harmful for the scalp, but the focus is on getting the paste on the individual strands of hair.)

3. Sweep the coated hair up on top of your head and cover with a plastic bag, securing with a hair clip or clothespin.

4. Leave on for 20 to 30 minutes.

5. Remove plastic bag and rinse the mixture off hair thoroughly using cool water. (Hot water will make the flour stick to the hair shafts.)

6. Shampoo as usual, rinsing with cool water.

HERBAL HAIR RINSES

Hair rinses are helpful in correcting hair's pH, removing residue from shampoo and other hair products, and creating a healthy-looking shine. Rinses can also bring out the highlights in your hair.

SHINY HAIR RINSE

Using apple cider vinegar and lemon juice is the best treatment for maintaining the natural pH balance of your hair and making it shiny. Omit the lemon juice and double the vinegar if you don't want even the slightest lightening of color.

Juice from ½ lemon
2 tablespoons (30 ml) apple cider vinegar
1 cup (250 ml) water

Yield: 1 treatment

To make:
1. Combine all ingredients in a pitcher or jar and mix well.
To use:
1. Shampoo and rinse hair as usual.
2. Pour the mixture on your hair and massage into the scalp and through the hair.
3. Rinse thoroughly with cool water.

BOUNCY HAIR RINSE

This one is so easy to make that anyone can do it — and there's no mixing involved. It's so effective that pretty soon everyone will be calling you Tigger — after Winnie-the-Pooh's bouncy friend!

1 cup (250 ml) beer

Yield: 1 treatment

To make:
1. Pour the beer into a glass and allow it to go flat and get warm.
To use:
1. Shampoo and rinse hair as usual.
2. Pour the flat warm beer on your hair and work it through.
3. Rinse thoroughly with cool water.

DEODORIZING HAIR RINSE

Anyone who has had to clean an animal that has tangoed with a skunk knows this deodorizing trick. Let's hope the odors you'll be trying to remove won't be as strong as skunk! This is great for getting the smell of smoke from your hair.

1 cup (250 ml) tomato juice
2 teaspoons (10 ml) water

Yield: 1 treatment

To make:
1. Combine the tomato juice and water thoroughly in a jar or pitcher.

To use:
1. Shampoo and rinse hair as usual.
2. Pour the tomato juice mixture on your hair and work it through.
3. Rinse thoroughly with cool water.

DANDRUFF RINSE

Restoring the hair to its mildly acid pH can help to clear up dandruff. See a physician if you don't start to see results in 1 to 2 weeks.

1 cup (250 ml) apple cider vinegar
1 cup (250 ml) water
2 tablespoons (30 ml) fresh lemongrass
2 tablespoons (30 ml) fresh nettle
2 tablespoons (30 ml) fresh peppermint

Yield: 7 treatments (1 week)

To make:
1. In a saucepan, bring the apple cider vinegar and water to a boil.
2. Place the herbs in a widemouthed jar.
3. Pour the boiling vinegar and water over the herbs.
4. Cover and steep for 1 week, shaking daily.
5. Strain out the herbs and decant the liquid.

To use:
1. Dilute ¼ cup (50 ml) herbal vinegar mixture with 1 cup (250 ml) water.
2. After shampooing and rinsing hair thoroughly, rinse with diluted vinegar.
3. Let the vinegar sit on the scalp for 1 minute.
4. Rinse thoroughly with cool water.
5. Pat hair dry.

OILY HAIR RINSE

Get out your field guide to gather the material for this one. Wild watercress is delicious to eat and full of vitamins and minerals that are good for the hair. This slightly acid rinse removes residue on the hair, leaving it squeaky clean. Found growing near or in stream and creek beds, watercress is abundant in the Northeast and elsewhere in the United States. You can also purchase it in most grocery stores.

⅔ cup (150 ml) water
1 teaspoon (5 ml) apple cider vinegar
2 cups (500 ml) fresh watercress (wild or cultivated)

Yield: 1 treatment

To make:

1. In a saucepan, warm the water and vinegar.
2. Rinse the watercress, removing any dirt and frayed leaves.
3. Place the watercress in a blender, then pour the warm vinegar water over the herbs.
4. Blend on high speed for 2 minutes.
5. Strain, reserving the liquid.

To use:

1. Use this rinse freshly made, while still warm; the heat helps it work.
2. Shampoo your hair, then rinse well.
3. While hair is still damp, pour the warm mixture onto the hair and scalp.
4. Leave on for 10 minutes.
5. Rinse with cool water.

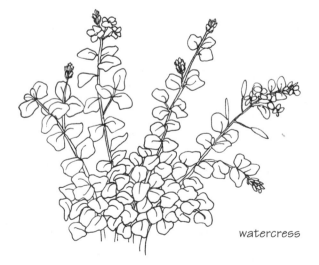

watercress

HERBAL SCALP TREATMENTS

Scalp treatments can rescue damaged hair and solve scalp problems such as dandruff and itchy scalp. Even if you do not have scalp problems, performing an herbal scalp treatment on a monthly basis can result in healthier, more manageable hair and a really clean, invigorated scalp.

OLIVE OIL TREATMENT

Olive oil conditions and improves the strength and elasticity of your hair, so it is a good addition to your shampoo. As a conditioning scalp treatment, the olive oil nourishes new hair. You may substitute other essential oils as you wish.

½ cup (125 ml) olive oil

5 drops frankincense essential oil

5 drops blue chamomile essential oil (optional)

1 plastic bag that can fit over your hair

Yield: 1 or 2 treatments, depending on hair length and thickness

To make:

1. Pour olive oil into a lotion jar, then add the essential oil.

2. Put on lid and shake well to disperse the essential oil.

3. Let sit for 24 hours in a cool, dark place. Shake again before use.

To use:

1. Rinse hair with warm water.

2. Warm 1 tablespoon (15 ml) of the oil in the palms of your hands.

3. Using your fingertips (not nails), gently massage the oil into the scalp in a circular motion.

4. Repeat until the entire scalp has been massaged.

5. Rub the ends of your hair with the remaining oil.

6. Place a plastic bag over your hair, secure by tying or with a hair clip or clothespin, and allow the oil to remain for at least ½ hour.

7. Rinse well, then shampoo as usual.

HERBAL STEAM

Similar to a facial steam, this treatment encourages circulation around the scalp and promotes healthy hair growth. Steam baths are beneficial for the whole body, but if you don't have one of them, this treatment is a great substitute. If your scalp starts to itch a little, don't worry; this is normal. Your skin is reacting to the increased circulation. When you do a scalp steam weekly, you'll find that the itching sensation gradually fades.

2 quarts (2 liters)
    water
2 teaspoons (10 ml)
    dried basil
2 teaspoons (10 ml)
    dried rose petals
2 teaspoons (10 ml)
    dried lavender
    petals
2 teaspoons (10 ml)
    dried lemon balm
2 teaspoons (10 ml)
    dried comfrey

Yield: 1 treatment

To make:
1. Bring water to a boil in a large stainless-steel or enamel spaghetti-type pot.
2. Add the dried herbs to the boiling water, cover, and turn off the heat.
3. After 2 minutes, uncover, give the herbs a stir, and remove from the stove.

To use:
1. Place the steaming pot on the floor at the end of your sofa or bed, positioning it so you can lie comfortably with your head 6 to 10 inches above the pot.
2. Loosely pin up your hair, allowing the steam to get to the scalp.
3. Drape a large towel around your hairline and let it hang down around the pot so that it catches the vapors and steam.
4. Keeping your head a comfortable distance from the pot, stay under the towel as long as you comfortably can.

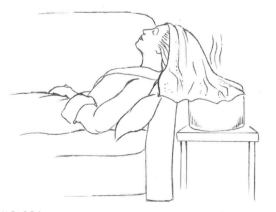

FLOWER ESSENCE SCALP MASSAGE

~~~~~~

Flower essences can work wonders to calm the nerves and soothe anyone who is stressed out. The essences are subtle healing substances extracted from flowers. Edward Bach developed a procedure for extracting the essences in the early 1900s. Rescue Remedy, the most popular, is actually a combination of five flower essences and is available in most health food stores. Incorporating flower essences into a scalp treatment benefits both the hair and the emotional and mental state of the recipient. This treatment, which is offered at finer spas, is remarkably easy to make and enjoy at home.

½ cup (125 ml) apricot kernel oil

3 drops red clover flower essence
3 drops lavender flower essence
or
3 drops Rescue Remedy flower essence (or other flower essence combination of your choice)
3 drops lavender essential oil

1 plastic bag that will fit over your hair

Yield: 1 treatment

To make:
1. First add the apricot kernel oil, then the flower essences and essential oils, to a lotion jar.
2. Shake well to disperse all ingredients.
3. Let sit for 24 hours in a cool, dark place; shake again before use.

To use:
1. Rinse hair with warm water.
2. Warm 1 tablespoon (15 ml) of the oil in the palms of your hands.
3. Using your fingertips (not nails), in a circular motion gently massage the oil into the scalp.
4. Repeat until the entire scalp has been massaged.
5. Rub the shafts and ends of your hair with the remaining oil.
6. Place a plastic bag over your hair, secure with a hair clip or clothespin, and allow the oil to remain for at least ½ hour.
7. Rinse well, then shampoo as you normally would.

DANDRUFF OIL TREATMENT

In treating dandruff, it is important to use an oil treatment for the scalp once each week. The olive oil treatment (see page 67) may be helpful, or try the following. The apple cider vinegar helps to balance the pH of your scalp and the cornmeal gently exfoliates the dry, flaky skin.

½ cup (125 ml) grape-
  seed oil
2 tablespoons (30
  ml) cornmeal
1 tablespoon (15 ml)
  apple cider vinegar
1 plastic bag that will
  fit over your hair

Yield: 1 or 2 treatments, depending on hair length and thickness

To make:
1. Pour the grapeseed oil into a bowl, then add the cornmeal and vinegar.
2. Stir well to make a pasty oil.
To use:
1. Rinse hair with warm water.
2. Warm a tablespoon of the oil mixture in the palms of your hands.
3. Using your fingertips (not nails), in a circular motion gently massage the mixture into the scalp.
4. Repeat until the entire scalp has been massaged.
5. Place a plastic bag over your hair, secure with a hair clip or clothespin, and allow the oil to remain for at least ½ hour.
6. Rinse well, then shampoo as you normally would.

ST.-JOHN'S-WORT AND BASIL OIL SCALP MASSAGE

St.-John's-wort is often used on burns, since it has properties that help regenerate damaged nerves. It is also recommended for stimulating new hair growth for people whose hair has been affected by radiation treatments, pulling, or other damage to the scalp. Basil also encourages hair growth.

Make this oil in midsummer, when the plants are in bloom; it is the flowers that hold the healing powers. The yellow flower and the leaves will turn the oil red. You may also purchase ready-made oil at a health food store.

2 cups (500 ml) fresh St.-John's-wort herb
1 cup (250 ml) fresh basil
3 cups (750 ml) olive oil
10 drops vitamin E oil
5 drops basil essential oil

Yield: 12 applications

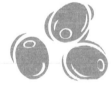

To make:

1. Gather the St.-John's-wort in midmorning, when the top of the plant is flowering. Gather the basil before it flowers.

2. Spread the herbs on paper towels and allow to wilt overnight.

3. Stuff the wilted herbs into a large glass jar, packing it as full as possible.

4. Pour the olive oil over the herbs, filling the jar to within ½" of the top.

5. Use a chopstick to poke the herbs and release any captured air or gases.

6. Top off with oil as necessary and screw on the lid of the jar.

7. Store the oil in a dark, cool spot.

8. Repeat steps 5, 6, and 7 daily for 6 days.

9. Let sit for another 6 days; on the 7th day, again repeat steps 5, 6, and 7.

10. Again, let sit for the next 6 days, then on the 7th day repeat steps 5, 6, and 7 again.

11. Let sit for the following 6 days, then strain the herbal material out of the oil and discard it, preserving your oil.

12. Add the vitamin E and basil essential oil to the St.-John's-wort and basil oil mixture, then store in an amber bottle.

To use:

1. Pour 2 tablespoons (30 ml) into a small dish.

2. Dip your fingertips (not nails) into bowl.

3. Gently massage the oil all over your scalp, working in a circular motion.

4. Allow the oil to stay on the scalp for at least ½ hour, then shampoo as you normally would.

5. Repeat a few times a week or even every day, if desired.

NATURAL HERBAL HAIR COLORING

Unlike many commercial hair coloring products that damage hair, herbal hair coloring products often condition the hair. So much so, in fact, many people choose to use neutral hennas for their conditioning properties.

FOR BLOND HAIR: LIGHTENING FORMULA

This formula is very effective when applied to light hair shades, but the darker your hair, the harder it will be to lighten it naturally. Persistence is the key. Use this treatment for several sunny days in a row and you're sure to see results.

⅓ cup (75 ml) water
3 tablespoons (45 ml) fresh chamomile flowers
3 tablespoons (45 ml) fresh calendula flowers
Juice from 3 lemons
Broad-brimmed straw hat (an old or inexpensive one that can be cut)
Long white cotton scarf or foot-wide strip of a bedsheet

Yield: 1–2 treatments

To make:
1. Bring the water to a boil.
2. Pour the boiling water over the fresh herbs and let steep for 20 minutes.
3. Strain the infusion, reserving the liquid.
4. Add the lemon juice and mix well.
5. Decant into a spray bottle.

To use:
1. For best results, pick a sunny day to do this treatment.
2. Cut out the top of your broad-brimmed hat. *Note:* If you have short hair, you will not need to use a hat.

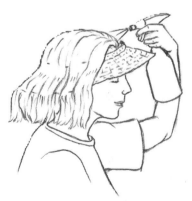

3. Put on the hat. Pull all your hair through the top, letting it spill down over the brim. If necessary, secure the hat using the scarf or bedsheet around the brim. The scarf can also help keep the lemon mixture from dripping down your face.

4. Spray the lemon mixture to thoroughly dampen all your hair.

5. Sit out in the sunshine (be sure to apply protection to other areas of your body). The longer you sit in the sun, the more lightening will occur; try at least ½ hour and up to 4 hours.

6. As your hair dries, repeat the lemon spray often.

7. Be sure to use a good conditioner — the olive oil or jojoba, for example — after using this treatment, as it tends to be drying.

BLOND HIGHLIGHTING RINSE

The effects of this rinse are subtle. The more you use it, the better the results.

Juice of 1 lemon
¼ cup (50 ml) water

Yield: 1 treatment

To make:

1. Place the lemon juice and water in a glass jar.

2. Shake well.

To use:

1. Shampoo and rinse your hair as usual.

2. Pour the lemon mixture into your hair.

3. Let sit for 5 minutes.

4. Rinse with cool water.

RED HIGHLIGHTING RINSE

1 cup (250 ml) water
1 tablespoon (15 ml)
   alkanet root

Yield: 1 treatment

To make:

1. Bring the water to a boil.

2. Place the alkanet root in a glass jar.

3. Pour the boiling water over the alkanet root.

4. Cover and steep for 10 minutes.

5. Strain root from infusion.

To use:

1. Shampoo and rinse hair as usual.

2. Pour the alkanet infusion into your hair, catching the liquid in a basin. Repour the infusion through the hair 10 times.

3. Let your hair sit for 5 minutes.

4. Rinse with cool water.

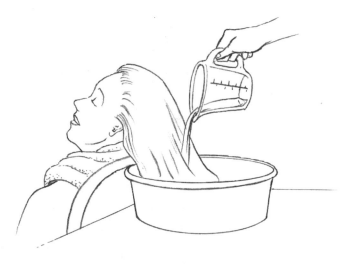

DARKENING HAIR RINSE

1 cup (250 ml) black
  walnut hulls
10 grape leaves
1 cup (250 ml) wine
1 cup (250 ml) water
Cast-iron Dutch oven

Yield: 1 treatment

To make:

1. Place the walnut hulls and grape leaves into the cast-iron Dutch oven.

2. Pour the wine and water over the herbs.

3. Simmer over low heat for 1 hour.

4. Strain, reserving the liquid.

To use:

1. Shampoo and rinse hair as usual.

2. Pour the herbal decoction into your hair, catching the liquid in a basin. Repour the infusion through your hair 10 times.

3. Wait 5 minutes.

4. Rinse with cool water.

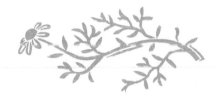

¼ cup dried calendula
flowers
½ cup (125 ml) red
henna
⅓ cup (75 ml) boiling
water
Rubber gloves
Plastic bag large
enough to fit over
hair and scalp

Yield: 1 treatment

To make:

1. In a spice mill, powder the calendula petals.

2. Sift together the henna and powdered calendula into a glass or porcelain bowl. (Do not use metal bowls or spoons with henna; the metal will affect the color.)

3. Pour the boiling water over the henna.

4. Mix thoroughly to form a thick paste.

To use:

1. Shampoo and rinse your hair as usual.

2. Wearing rubber gloves, use a wooden or plastic spoon to apply the henna to your hair. Try to avoid getting the henna mixture on your scalp.

3. Still wearing rubber gloves, once the entire head of hair is covered with the henna mixture, massage the henna into your hair to the ends.

4. Wrap the hair on top of your head and cover the hair with the plastic bag, securing it with a hair clip or clothespin.

5. Immediately, using soap, wash off any henna that may have dripped down your face or gotten on your hands or clothing.

6. Let the henna set for 20 to 40 minutes.

7. Rinse your hair thoroughly with warm water until the water runs clear.

8. Shampoo as usual, rinsing well with cool water.

NOTE ON APPLYING HENNA

When applying henna, avoid getting the coloring on your scalp. It will stain the scalp quite heavily. It is inevitable that some henna will get on your scalp, but the less of it, the better. Henna on the scalp will eventually wash out with shampooing, but it's best to minimize the problem by not rubbing any henna mixture into the scalp.

FOR BRUNET HAIR: SHADES OF BROWN

There are many henna color choices available these days. Shop around until you find a store with a good selection. You can use just one henna color for this treatment, or mix several shades. Henna will make your hair redder or browner, but not lighter.

2 tablespoons (30 ml) powdered cloves

2 tablespoons (30 ml) quassia bark

½ cup (125 ml) brown henna

⅓ cup (75 ml) boiling water

Rubber gloves

Plastic bag large enough to fit over hair and scalp

Yield: 1 treatment

To make:

1. In a spice mill, powder the cloves and quassia bark.

2. Sift the henna, powdered cloves, and quassia bark together into a glass or porcelain bowl. (Do not use metal bowls or spoons with henna; metal affects the color.)

3. Pour the boiling water over the henna.

4. Mix thoroughly to form a thick paste.

To use:

1. Shampoo and rinse your hair as usual.

2. Wearing rubber gloves, use a wooden or plastic spoon to apply the henna to your hair. Try to avoid getting too much of the mixture on your scalp.

3. Once the entire head of hair is covered with the henna mixture, and still wearing rubber gloves, massage the henna into the hair all the way to the ends.

4. Wrap the hair on top of your head and cover the hair with the plastic bag, securing with a hair clip or clothespin.

5. Immediately, with soap, wash off any henna that may have dripped down your face or gotten on your hands or clothing.

6. Let the henna set on your hair for 20 to 40 minutes.

7. Rinse your hair thoroughly with warm water until the water runs clear.

8. Shampoo as usual, rinsing well with cool water.

FOR VERY DARK HAIR: SHADES OF BLACK

For very dark hair, you can substitute black henna for brown henna in the preceding brunet recipe, or try the following formula.

⅓ cup (75 ml) dried indigo

⅓ cup (75 ml) dried lavender

⅓ cup (75 ml) dried black malva flowers

⅓ cup (75 ml) boiling water

Rubber gloves

Plastic bag large enough to fit over hair and scalp

Yield: 1 treatment

To make:

1. In a spice mill, powder the dried herbs.

2. Sift the powdered herbs together into a glass or porcelain bowl. (Do not use metal bowls or spoons; metal affects the color.)

3. Pour the boiling water over the powdered herbs.

4. Mix thoroughly to form a thick paste.

To use:

1. Shampoo and rinse your hair as usual.

2. Wearing rubber gloves, use a wooden or plastic spoon to apply the mixture to your hair. Try to avoid getting the henna mixture on your scalp.

3. Once your entire head of hair is covered with the mixture, massage it into the hair to the ends.

4. Wrap the hair on top of your head and cover the hair with the plastic bag.

5. Immediately, using soap, wash off any herbal paste that may have dripped down your face or gotten on your hands or clothing.

6. Let the mixture set for 30 to 60 minutes.

7. Rinse your hair thoroughly with warm water, until the water runs clear.

8. Shampoo as usual, rinsing well with cool water.

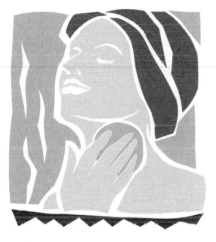

Herbal Rituals for a Beautiful Face and Neck

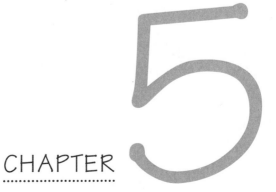

CHAPTER

If the eyes are the windows of the soul, then the face is the reflection of the physical being. Facial treatments and skin care have a great impact on your overall appearance and the health of your skin. In this chapter, you'll learn about creating your own facial rituals at home. This is not to say that you won't ever want to get a professional facial; you may. But you'll see how easy it can be to do facial steams without fancy, expensive equipment. You may also be surprised to find a plethora of ingredients for facial scrubs and masks in your kitchen right now, without even going to the grocery store.

Once you begin making the recipes in this chapter, the only lotions or skin creams you'll need to buy will be for sunscreen purposes, although you can try your hand at making those yourself, as well (see chapter 11). The ritual of creating floral waters may become an enjoyable part of your life, as may the process of creating astringents, face washes, and even after-shaves for all members of your family.

HERBAL EYE TREATMENTS

The eyes are the most delicate area on your face. They are also its focal point, and it's important to treat your eyes tenderly. Eye packs are easy applications to combine with other treatments such as a foot massage and a body wrap.

APPLYING EYE TREATMENT

In applying creams, lotions, and eye makeup, it's worth taking a bit of extra care so that you keep the skin around your eyes looking as healthy as possible. Following are the application steps I suggest:

1. Dab the product of choice onto your ring finger.
2. Gently pat the lotion, under the eye, starting at the outside and working in.
3. Next pat the lotion on top of the eye, again starting at the outside and working in.

Note: Working in the other direction, from inside to outside, encourages crow's-feet wrinkles.

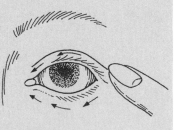

VIOLET EYE CREAM

Tired of spending a fortune on eye creams? This recipe is great for tired, puffy, or irritated eyes — or just for day-to-day makeup removal. This exquisite formula is very popular; as a matter of fact, I just made 24 jars of cream for my dear friend Maria. The blue chamomile essential oil is expensive (approximately $50 for ½ ounce). It's high in azulene — an anti-inflammatory agent extracted from chamomile flowers — and it's very soothing to the delicate area around the eye. It's not crucial for the recipe, but a great addition when you can afford the indulgence. If you are allergic to chamomile tea, leave it out.

½ cup (125 ml) fresh violet flowers

½ cup (125 ml) fresh violet leaves

1¼ cups (300 ml) almond oil

½ cup (125 ml) fresh horsetail

2 tablespoons (30 ml) beeswax

10 drops vitamin E oil

10 drops blue chamomile essential oil (optional)

Yield: Approximately 30 ¼-ounce containers

To make:

1. Gather the violet leaves and flowers and place them on a towel to wilt overnight.

2. In a double boiler, steep the leaves, petals, and horsetail in oil over low heat for 5 hours.

3. Grate the beeswax or cut into small pieces.

4. Strain the plant material from the oil completely.

5. Pour the oil back into the double boiler, adding the grated beeswax.

6. Melt the beeswax into the oil completely, then remove from heat.

7. Quickly add the vitamin E and blue chamomile oils.

8. Pour into dainty ¼-ounce (7-g) containers or jars.

9. Decorate with violet stickers.

To use, refer to Applying Eye Treatment box.

BE SELECTIVE ABOUT YOUR UTENSILS

In all your herbal preparations, the type of cooking utensils you use is important. Use nonreactive utensils made of stainless steel, glass, or enamel. Do not use aluminum, copper, or cast iron; these metals will affect the finished product.

CUCUMBER EYE PACK

Cucumbers have long been known to sooth puffy eyes. We've all seen in magazines the models with cucumbers on their eyes, so what's the hesitation? It doesn't get much easier than this!

¼ cucumber

Yield: 1 treatment

To make:
1. Slice the cucumber to fit over eyes.
2. If you really like things simple, cut just two slices. I prefer to slice 5 to 10 extremely thin slices and use several on each eye. Either method works.

To use:
1. Spritz eye area with water.
2. Lying down, place cucumber slices on your eyelids and leave in place for 5–10 minutes.

BAGGY EYE TREATMENT

Raw potato slices will help tighten baggy, puffy eyes. All you need is a potato and a knife or slicer!

¼ potato

Yield: 1 treatment

To make:
1. Slice the potato to fit over your eyes.
2. Cut 2 slices, or, if you prefer, 5 to 10 very thin slices, several for each eye. Either method works.

To use:
1. Spritz eye area with water.
2. Lying down, place the potato slices on your eyelids and leave in place for at least 10 minutes for best results.

CROW'S-FEET TREATMENT

Here's another treatment that's easy to whip up! Egg whites help plump and firm wrinkled skin.

1 egg white
Cotton ball

Yield: 1 treatment

To make:
1. Beat the egg white to just before it forms soft peaks.
To use:
1. Dab the egg white in a crescent shape around the eye, along the cheekbone and the outer eye area.
2. Allow to sit for 10 minutes.
3. Spritz the egg white with water.
4. Using cool water on a cotton ball, gently remove.

HERBAL EYELASH AND BROW TREATMENTS

The eyelashes and brows, like any hairs on your body, respond to the moisturizing effects of natural oils. Pampering these eye hairs makes them healthier and more manageable, and bolder looking without the need for mascara or brow pencil.

NOURISHING OIL

Castor bean oil is nourishing for the eyelashes and brows. If you are sensitive to mascara, as I am, this recipe is a good substitute for accentuating the natural color of your lashes. You can use this application daily, and once applied, it can be left on all day.

1 teaspoon (5 ml)
   castor bean oil
Cotton swab

Yield: 1 treatment

To use:
1. Dab the cotton swab into the oil and apply to the lashes only, being careful not to get any oil on the skin surrounding the eye.
2. Dab the eyebrow where it is most thickly haired.
3. Using your ring finger, gently rub the oil over the entire eyebrow.

HERBAL EYE PILLOW

This little eye pillow blocks light and provides slight weight and pressure, which will relax the eyes and facial muscles, thus reducing tension, stimulating circulation, and relieving mild headaches. If you have a sewing machine and can stitch a straight seam, you can easily make your own version that matches any store-bought ones. You can wash the cover without having to clean the entire pillow.

¼ yard (23 cm) silky, natural, washable fabric (silk or cotton is best)

1 cup (250 ml) flaxseed

½ cup (125 ml) lavender flowers

3 drops essential oil of lavender (optional)

Yield: One eye pillow

To make:

1. Choose a fabric in a color that is soothing to you.

2. Fold the fabric in half, right sides together, and trace the eye pillow and cover patterns (see appendix, page 193) onto the wrong side of the fabric. Cut on the lines.

3. With right sides together, stitch a ½" (1¼ cm) seam around the long sides and one end of the pillow. Turn right side out. Stitch the two long sides, and one short end of the cover as well. Hem the edges of the open end by hand or machine.

4. Mix the lavender and flaxseed (adding the scent, if desired).

5. Stuff the pillow with the flower and seed mixture.

6. Hand-sew the remaining side closure.

To use:

1. Squeeze the lavender and flaxseed in the eye pillow to release the soothing lavender scent.

2. Place the eye pillow in the washable cover.

3. Place over the eyes while relaxing or receiving another treatment.

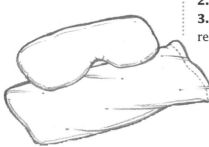

HERBAL LIP TREATMENTS

Do you know someone who seems "addicted" to a commercial lip treatment product? The product may contain chemicals that are irritating to the lips, encouraging continued use of the product. To avoid commercial lip balm addictions, make your own pure, simple products that you will be free to use as needed.

LIP BALM

These are a snap to make, and the recipe lends itself to numerous variations. Use an infused oil to incorporate the healing properties of herbs into your balm (see page 107). Pam Montgomery taught me this basic recipe, which we made green in our apprenticeship class. I prefer to add the alkanet, which yields a range of shades from red to pink to spicy and also adds emollient benefits. It's a great project to do with children; let each one choose a pretty sticker to decorate the dainty container. These make great party favors, too.

½ cup (125 ml) oil (apricot kernel, almond, or grapeseed)
2 tablespoons (30 ml) grated beeswax
½ teaspoon (2½ ml) alkanet root
10 drops natural flavoring oil
3 drops vitamin E oil
Stickers

Yield: Approximately 15 ¼-ounce (7-gram) containers

LIP BALM RECIPE VARIATIONS

Banana. Omit alkanet root and use banana flavoring oil.

Cinnamon. Use an oil infused with plantain and comfrey and add cinnamon flavoring.

Cherry Red. Double the amount of alkanet root for a deep red color and add cherry flavoring.

Use your imagination and develop your own variations.

To make:

1. In a double boiler, gently heat oil to melt the beeswax.

2. Add enough alkanet root for desired redness. (Oil should look black for a deep red color and red for a lighter shade.)

3. When beeswax is entirely melted, strain the oil into an easy-pour measuring cup, removing the alkanet root from the mix.

4. Add the natural flavoring oil and vitamin E and pour into containers.

LIP WRINKLE WONDER

Papaya is great for diminishing wrinkles around the lips.

¼ very ripe papaya **or** ¼ cup (50 ml) papaya juice

Yield: 1 treatment

To make:
1. Mash the papaya into a mushy pulp.
To use:
1. Lie down with a towel behind your head and your hair pulled back.
2. Generously apply the papaya mush to your lips and the surrounding area. If you are using juice, apply to a cotton ball and dab the area around your lips. (This is also great for breakout-prone areas such as the T-zone.)
3. Leave on for 10 minutes; follow with a facial exfoliation treatment (see pages 92–95).
4. Rinse with cool water.

DAILY CLEANSERS

These gentle products are great for daily use and a fresh, clean feel. The following recipes were inspired by and adapted from Connie Krochmal's *Natural Cosmetics from Beehive to Herb Garden.*

HERBAL CLEANSING MILK FOR DRY SKIN

2 tablespoons (30 ml) dried chamomile blossoms
2 tablespoons (30 ml) dried rose petals
2 tablespoons (30 ml) dried lemon balm
2 tablespoons (30 ml) dried calendula
2 tablespoons (30 ml) dried comfrey
1 tablespoon (15 ml) bee pollen

1 cup (250 ml) boiling water
¼ cup (50 ml) aloe vera gel
½ cup (125 ml) glycerin
2 tablespoons (30 ml) honey
10 drops vitamin E oil
Yield: 4 treatments

To make:
1. Place the dried flowers and herbs and bee pollen in a 10-ounce (284-gram) glass jar with lid.
2. Pour the boiling water over the flowers and pollen, cover, and steep for 20 minutes.

3. Strain out herbs, reserving the liquid.

4. Pour the liquid into a blender and add the remaining ingredients.

5. Blend at high speed for 2 minutes.

6. Pour into a widemouthed jar.

7. Keep refrigerated; mixture will last 1 week.

APPLYING FACIAL CLEANSERS

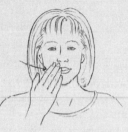
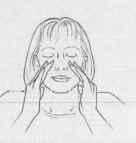

1. Apply cleanser to the throat using gentle strokes across the neck from side to side, starting at the upper shoulders and moving up.

2. Apply to the face with a side-to-side motion, gently swiping across the chin, above the lips, and then across the forehead.

3. Using your fingertips, gently massage in upward strokes. Start at the jaw outside the mouth, coming up along the side of the nose and across the bridge of the nose.

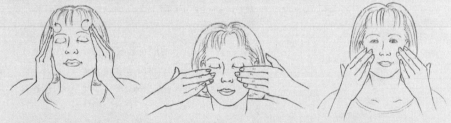

4. Make several spiraling, circular motions spanning the entire forehead, ending up above and outside the eyes.

5. Press the cheekbones with very light pressure, moving from the outer side inward.

6. Use a spiral, circular stroke on the cheeks.

Repeat steps 1 through 6. Using a warm facecloth (or a diaper!), cover your entire face and gently dab all over. Rinse with cool water.

HERBAL CLEANSING MILK FOR NORMAL SKIN

2 tablespoons (30 ml) dried elder flower blossoms

2 tablespoons (30 ml) dried rose petals

2 tablespoons (30 ml) dried lavender

2 tablespoons (30 ml) dried calendula

2 tablespoons (30 ml) dried comfrey

1 tablespoon (15 ml) bee pollen

1 cup (250 ml) boiling water

¼ cup (50 ml) aloe vera gel

¼ cup (50 ml) glycerin

¼ cup (50 ml) honey

10 drops vitamin E oil

Yield: 4 treatments

To make:

1. Place the dried herbs and flowers and bee pollen in a 10-ounce (284-gram) glass jar with lid.

2. Pour the boiling water over the flowers and pollen; cover and steep for 20 minutes.

3. Strain, reserving the liquid.

4. Pour the liquid into a blender and add the remaining ingredients.

5. Blend at high speed for 2 minutes.

6. Pour into a widemouthed jar.

7. Keep refrigerated; mixture will last 1 week.

To use, refer to the Applying Facial Cleansers box.

HERBAL CLEANSING GEL FOR OILY SKIN

2 tablespoons (30 ml) dried parsley

2 tablespoons (30 ml) dried rose petals

2 tablespoons (30 ml) dried rosemary

2 tablespoons (30 ml) dried calendula

2 tablespoons (30 ml) dried linden blossoms

1 cup (250 ml) boiling water

½ cup (125 ml) aloe vera gel

¼ tablespoon (4 ml) honey

10 drops vitamin E oil

Yield: 4 treatments

To make:

1. Place the dried flowers and herbs in a 10-ounce (284-gram) glass jar with lid.

2. Pour the boiling water over the flowers; cover and steep for 20 minutes.

3. Strain, reserving the liquid.

4. Pour the liquid into a blender and add the remaining ingredients.

5. Blend at high speed for 2 minutes.

6. Pour into a widemouthed jar.

7. Keep refrigerated; mixture will last 1 week.

To use, refer to the Applying Facial Cleansers box.

FACIAL STEAMS

How do you think those movie stars stay so beautiful? Well, you say you want movie-star results but you don't have a movie-star budget? Don't fret. You don't need any fancy equipment to hydrate your face — just a large pot of water, a big towel, and a selection of herbs. Receiving a facial in a salon is a wonderful treat, but you don't have to wait for an appointment when you do it at home. These treatments are very easy.

Many students of aesthetics have told me what a difference they noted in their skin after serving as facial steam guinea pigs in classes over the course of a semester. Facial steams are recommended on a weekly basis.

BASIC HERBAL FACIAL STEAM

You may find that your face gets itchy the first time you steam it. This is normal; your skin is reacting to the increased circulation caused by the steam. If you give yourself a facial steam weekly, you'll find that the itching sensation will decrease gradually, and the increased circulation will have your face all aglow.

2 quarts (2 liters) water
1 cup (250 ml) dried herbs
Large spaghetti-type pot

Yield: 1 treatment

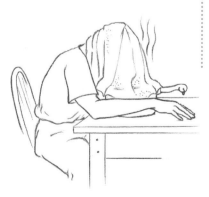

To make:
1. Bring water to a boil in a large pot.
2. Add dried herb mixture to the boiling water, cover, and turn off the heat.
3. After 2 minutes, uncover, give the herbs a stir, and remove from the stove.
To use:
1. Place the pot on a table or counter where you can sit comfortably with your face about 6 inches above it. Drape a large towel over your head and allow it to hang down around the pot so that it catches the vapors and steam.
2. Keeping a comfortable distance from the pot, try to stay under the towel as long as you comfortably can.

HERBAL FACE LIFT

Remember this recipe the next time you're getting ready to go to your high school reunion! It's very effective at tightening the skin under the chin and the neck and can also reduce some of the roundness in your cheeks. This recipe is too drying for the eye area, which has no oil ducts; avoid applying it there. Use Violet Eye Cream (see recipe on page 81) to plump up the skin around the eyes.

½ cup (125 ml) baking soda
½ cup (125 ml) orrisroot
¼ cup (50 ml) sea salt
2 tablespoons (30 ml) dulse
2 tablespoons (30 ml) kelp
½ cup (125 ml) distilled water
Several strips of 8" by 8' (20 cm by 2.4 m) torn bedsheets, gauze, or other clean cotton material

Yield: 1 treatment

To make:

1. Sift together the baking soda, orrisroot, and sea salt into a large bowl.

2. In a spice mill, powder the dulse and kelp and add to the dry ingredients.

3. Heat the distilled water to boiling, then pour over the dry ingredients.

4. Stir thoroughly.

To use:

1. Wear a shirt with a fairly low neckline for easy access to your neck and chin.

2. Moisturize the jaw, chin, neck, and cheek area of your face with a light moisturizer or vegetable oil. Dab your face with a cloth to remove any excess oil or moisturizer.

3. Using a wooden spoon, apply the mixture to the jaw, chin, neck, and cheeks.

FACIAL STEAM HERB SUGGESTIONS

Use any of the herbs listed for your skin type, or a combination.

Dry skin: rose, lavender, comfrey, chamomile

Normal skin: rose, lavender, lemon balm, calendula

Oily skin: rosemary, sage, witch hazel

Problem (dull or breakout-prone) skin: comfrey

4. Immediately wrap the sheets or gauze snuggly first around the neck, then from the chin around the head several times, to just below the eyes. Next, wrap sheet or gauze up over top of head and under the chin a few times to secure. I like to combine this treatment with the cucumber eye treatment. Another option is to soak cotton balls in floral water or a natural oil and to place them on the closed eyelids.

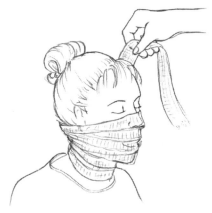

5. Relax and be quiet until the mixture and sheets become dry and tight (approximately 30 minutes). No talking — this will stretch the sheets and keep you from getting the results you desire.

6. Rinse your face and neck with the coldest water you can bear. Notice the surprising softening effects on your skin.

PAPAYA ENZYME TREATMENT

This treatment is used in conjunction with a facial steam to help clear up blemishes.

1 very ripe papaya

Yield: 1 treatment

To make:
1. Mash the papaya into a mushy pulp.
To use:
1. Prepare a facial steam according to the recipe on page 89.
2. Generously apply the papaya mush to your face, being careful to avoid the eyes.
3. Steam your face with the papaya on it following the instructions for the facial steam.

HERBAL SCRUBS AND MASKS

Nuts and grains are popular ingredients in facial scrubs and masks. Aduki beans, oatmeal, barley, garbanzo beans, and even poppy seeds help to exfoliate the skin. Nuts are particularly good if you have dry skin because of their high fat content. Recipes for a few facial scrubs and masks follow, but again, please don't limit yourself to just these ingredients. If there is a commercial product you like, look at the ingredients and try your hand at creating a similar product at home — without the added chemical preservatives.

APPLYING FACIAL PRODUCTS

For best results and to minimize aging effects, apply products to the face by using upward and outward strokes. Apply products with your fingertips (not fingernails) in small, circular motions. Use only your ring finger anywhere near your eyes and use inward strokes. The eye area has the most delicate skin and the ring finger is the weakest finger, thus discouraging crow's feet.

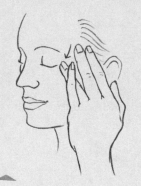

AVENA FACIAL GRAINS

These grains can be packaged in a pretty glass spice jar with a shaker top. Decorate with stickers and ribbon for a beautiful gift. This recipe was inspired by Rosemary Gladstar's "Miracle Grains." I've used the oat bran and poppy seeds for gentle exfoliation. This recipe may be easily doubled for gift-giving.

½ cup (125 ml) oat-
  meal
¼ cup (50 ml) oat
  bran
3 tablespoons (45 ml)
  almonds
½ cup (125 ml) white
  clay
2 tablespoons (30 ml)
  poppy seeds
2 tablespoons (30 ml)
  dried herbs

Yield: 16 treatments

To make:

1. In a blender or spice/coffee mill, grind the oatmeal and oat bran, leaving some grit.
2. Grind the almonds and strain, leaving a bit of grit for exfoliation of the skin.
3. Combine with all other ingredients in a large bowl, using a wire whisk to mix.
4. Package in four 1-ounce spice jars.

To use:

1. Combine 1 tablespoon (15 ml) grains with 1 tablespoon (15 ml) water, milk, or yogurt and mix into a paste.
2. Apply to face by rubbing gently and in a circular motion. Especially treat the T-zone: This is the often oily area of the face that includes the forehead, nose, mouth, and chin (which form a T shape).
3. Rinse with warm water and then with cooler water.

HERBS FOR FACIAL GRAINS

Dry skin: rose, lavender

Normal skin: rose, lavender, lemon balm, calendula

Oily skin: rosemary, sage, witch hazel

Problem (dull or breakout-prone) skin: Use green clay instead of white and add 1 teaspoon (5 ml) goldenseal, 1 teaspoon (5 ml) myrrh, and 1 teaspoon (5 ml) comfrey root

OXYGEN FACIAL

This treatment is the latest rage at many top spas. The recipe contains hydrogen peroxide, which releases oxygen as it is combined with the other ingredients and applied to the skin. Oxygen helps slow the aging process. Be sure to make it fresh for best results.

⅛ cup (25 ml) oatmeal
1 tablespoon (15 ml) almonds
1 tablespoon (15 ml) white clay
1 teaspoon (5 ml) dried rose petals
1 tablespoon (15 ml) hydrogen peroxide
3 tablespoons (45 ml) water

Yield: 1 treatment

To make:

1. In a blender or spice/coffee mill, grind the oatmeal, leaving some grit.

2. Grind the almonds and strain, leaving a bit of grit for exfoliation of the skin.

3. Combine all dry ingredients in a large bowl, using a wire whisk to mix.

To use:

1. In a small bowl, combine the oatmeal mixture with the hydrogen peroxide and water, and form into a paste.

2. Apply to face by rubbing gently in a circular motion.

3. Allow to set on the face for 5 minutes.

4. Rinse with cool water.

HERBAL TREATMENTS FOR BLACKHEADS

Use this treatment in conjunction with the facial steam to help clear up blackheads.

¼ cup (50 ml) parsley

Yield: 1 treatment

To make:

1. Juice the parsley in a juicer or blender.

To use:

1. Prepare a facial steam according to the instructions on page 89.

2. Generously apply the parsley juice and pulp to the areas on your face that are prone to blackheads, avoiding the eyes.

3. Steam your face with the parsley juice on it, following the instructions for facial steams.

PEEL-OFF MASK

I bet you didn't think you could create one of these fancy masks at home. Good news! Since they contain primarily gelatin, herbal infusion, and juice, peel-off masks are quite simple to make. This recipe was inspired by and adapted from Janice Cox's *Natural Beauty at Home.*

¼ cup (50 ml) fruit juice
¼ cup (50 ml) herbal infusion (see page 142)
1 packet unflavored gelatin

Yield: 1 treatment

To make:
1. Pour the liquid ingredients into an oven-proof glass container.
2. Add the gelatin, stirring to dissolve completely.
3. Gently heat the mixture in a double boiler for 1 minute, stirring constantly.
4. Refrigerate the mixture for 30 minutes.

To use:
1. Spread a thin layer over your face and allow it to dry.
2. Peel off and rinse with cool water.
3. Pat dry.

JUICE AND HERBAL INFUSION SUGGESTIONS FOR PEEL-OFF MASK

Sensitive and fair skin: apple juice with rose petal infusion

Dry skin: honeydew or cantaloupe juice with lemon balm infusion

Normal skin: raspberry juice with raspberry leaf infusion

Oily skin: watermelon juice with rosemary infusion

Break-out-prone skin: tomato juice with garlic infusion

LOTIONS AND POTIONS

Many of us spend a fortune on face and body creams and lotions. The following recipes are exquisite and though they are a bit tricky, they are by far my most-sought-after products. I call them face creams, but they are affordable enough to make and use for your whole body. Although they do go on a little greasy, your skin will be hydrated by the pure vegetable ingredients, unlike many of the mineral oil products currently on the market. These moisturizers were inspired by Rosemary Gladstar's work; I hope you enjoy my modifications to the basic cream.

ROSE PINK FACE MOISTURIZER

This is my best-seller. You may omit the alkanet root if you don't want the pink color, although alkanet does offer some sunscreen protection. Everyone loves this recipe, but it's especially good for dry skin.

²/₃ cup (150 ml) grape-seed oil

¹/₃ cup (75 ml) coconut oil

1 teaspoon (5 ml) cocoa butter

1 tablespoon (15 ml) beeswax

¹/₂ teaspoon (2¹/₂ ml) alkanet root

¹/₃ cup (75 ml) rose water

¹/₃ cup (75 ml) distilled water

¹/₃ cup (75 ml) aloe vera gel

20 drops vitamin E oil

8 drops rose essential oil or attar of roses

15 1-ounce (25-gram) jars

Yield: Fifteen 1-ounce (25-gram) jars

To make:

1. In a double boiler, melt grapeseed oil, coconut oil, cocoa butter, beeswax, and alkanet root.

2. Once the beeswax is melted, strain out alkanet root and pour oil mixture into a glass measuring cup, preferably one with a spout.

3. Let cool to room temperature for approximately 1 hour.

4. Set up 15 clean jars on the edge of your counter for easy pouring.

5. Combine the rose water, distilled water, aloe vera gel, vitamin E, and essential oil in the blender and turn to the highest speed for a minute or two.

6. In a slow, thin drizzle, pour the cooled oils into the vortex of the waters while the blender is still going.

7. Listen to the blender; when it chokes, the water and oil have combined.

8. Pour into the jars and decorate with stickers and ribbons.

LAVENDER BLUE FACE MOISTURIZER

This cream contains blue chamomile essential oil, which adds a hint of color along with its healing and regenerative properties. Some people don't care for the scent of the blue chamomile, so smell it first. It is also quite expensive. Although it is very good for your skin, I would never recommend you use a scent that you find unpleasant. Frankincense essential oil also contributes regenerative properties.

⅔ cup (150 ml) grape-
    seed oil
⅓ cup (75 ml) coconut
    oil
1 teaspoon (5 ml)
    cocoa butter
1 tablespoon (30 ml)
    beeswax
⅓ cup ('75 ml) lavender
    water
⅓ cup (75 ml) distilled
    water
⅓ cup (75 ml) aloe
    vera gel
20 drops vitamin E oil
5 drops blue chamomile
    essential oil
5 drops lavender
    essential oil
5 drops frankincense
    essential oil
15 1-ounce (25-gram)
    jars

Yield: Fifteen 1-ounce (25-gram) jars

To make:

1. In a double boiler, melt the grapeseed oil, coconut oil, cocoa butter, and beeswax.
2. Once the beeswax is melted, pour the oil mixture into a glass measuring cup, preferably one with a spout.
3. Let cool to room temperature for approximately 1 hour.
4. Set up 15 clean jars on the edge of your counter for easy pouring.
5. Combine the lavender water, distilled water, aloe vera gel, vitamin E, and essential oils in the blender and turn to the highest speed for a minute or two.
6. In a slow, thin drizzle, pour the cooled oils into the vortex of the waters while the blender is still going.
7. Listen to the blender; when it chokes, the water and oil have combined.
8. Pour into the jars and decorate with stickers and ribbons.

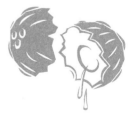

ORANGE BLOSSOM FACE CREAM

◄▼▼▼►

Emollient and hydrating, this is a cheery skin cream. The sesame oil in this recipe is a bit greasier than the grapeseed oil used in the other face cream recipes, and it has a stronger scent, but it adds sunscreen protection. Be sure to use cold pressed sesame oil, which will have a lighter scent than the toasted sesame oil found in the international cooking section of your local store. If you want added sunscreen protection, see the suggestions in chapter 11.

⅔ cup (150 ml) sesame oil

⅓ cup (75 ml) coconut oil

1 teaspoon (5 ml) cocoa butter

1 tablespoon (15 ml) beeswax

1 teaspoon (5 ml) alkanet root

3 tablespoons (45 ml) calendula

⅓ cup (75 ml) orange blossom water

⅓ cup (75 ml) distilled water

⅓ cup (75 ml) aloe vera gel

20 drops vitamin E oil

10 drops orange blossom essential oil

15 1-ounce (25-gram) jars

Yield: Fifteen 1-ounce (25-gram) jars

To make:

1. In a double boiler, melt the sesame oil, coconut oil, cocoa butter, beeswax, alkanet root, and calendula.

2. Once the beeswax is melted, strain out the alkanet root and pour the oil mixture into a glass measuring cup, preferably one with a spout.

3. Let cool to room temperature for approximately 1 hour.

4. Set up 15 clean jars on the edge of your counter for easy pouring.

5. Combine the orange blossom water, distilled water, aloe vera gel, vitamin E, and essential oil in the blender and turn to the highest speed for a minute or two.

6. In a slow, thin drizzle, pour the cooled oils into the vortex of the water while the blender is still going.

7. Listen to the blender; when it chokes, the water and oil have combined.

8. Pour in the jars and decorate with stickers and ribbons.

FLORAL WATERS

While you can buy aromatic floral waters (also called herbal waters or hydrosols), I find making my own to be an enchanting practice. Floral waters are distilled waters that are all natural and lightly scented. They are wonderful additions to any herbal product, especially moisturizing creams. Less concentrated then essential oils and therefore safe for use undiluted, hydrosols offer many of the same benefits as essential oils. You don't need a lot of sophisticated equipment to make floral waters at home. Once you figure out the arrangement of materials in this homemade "still," it all works almost effortlessly. I like to make floral waters when I plan to be working in the kitchen on something else. While I am preparing meals or other herbal preparations, I can keep an eye on the temperature of the herbal water and the ice and still get other things accomplished.

SUGGESTIONS FOR FLORAL WATERS

Any aromatic herbs will work in this venture. My favorites are rose, lavender, sage, marjoram, lemon balm, any of the mints, and lovage. Be creative!

- ◆ **For dry skin,** try rose and lavender.
- ◆ **For normal skin,** try lemon balm and mints.
- ◆ **For oily skin,** try sage, rosemary, and lovage.

AROMATIC FLORAL WATER

Large pot (12 to 16 quarts)

1 clean brick or flat rock

Bunch of fresh aromatic herbs or flowers (approximately ½ gallon or 2 pounds)

Glass bowl that fits down inside the pot (with 1" clearance around sides)

Water

Stainless-steel bowl large enough to sit on top of the large pot

1 large chunk of ice

Yield: Varies from 2 to 5 oz.

To make:

1. Place the large pot on the stove.

2. Place the brick in the center of the pot.

3. Arrange the fresh herbal material around the brick.

4. Add water up to the top of the brick. This will cover the herbs or flowers.

5. Place the glass bowl on top of the brick. This is where the distilled floral water will collect.

6. Set the stainless-steel bowl on top of the pot and add a large chunk of ice to the bowl. It is best to use one large chunk of ice created by filling a plastic jug with water and then freezing. Smaller ice cubes, while workable, tend to melt faster and require more attention than the big chunk.

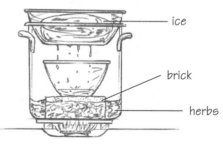

ice

brick

herbs

7. Turn the stove burner on low. Gently simmer the herbal mixture on the lowest heat (use a flame tamer if you have a gas range) for approximately 3 hours, taking care that there is always ice in the top. After 3 hours, remove the cover and enjoy the intoxicating aroma wafting through your home. The floral water will have collected in the glass bowl. Bottle this water in a capped container. Use it as a toner (especially good for dry skin) or an astringent, or add it to a face cream recipe.

HERBAL ASTRINGENTS AND AFTERSHAVES

Herbal astringents and aftershaves are used to tone the skin after cleansing. Many astringents contain floral waters and some sort of alcohol, both of which balance the pH of the skin and remove impurities.

QUEEN OF HUNGARY WATER

This recipe was developed for the Queen of Hungary in 1370. It's a wonderful astringent for those with normal, oily, or problem skin, and it's especially good for people with itchy skin. It's touted as the first herbal product to be produced and marketed. Although I include it with astringents, it was used by the Gypsies for almost everything you can think of, from mouthwash to hair rinse to footbaths. I like to use it in the bath. This recipe is best made with fresh herbs.

5 tablespoons (75 ml) fresh lemon balm

4 tablespoons (60 ml) fresh roses

4 tablespoons (60 ml) fresh chamomile

3 tablespoons (45 ml) fresh calendula

3 tablespoons (45 ml) fresh comfrey

1 tablespoon (15 ml) fresh lemon peel

1 tablespoon (15 ml) fresh rosemary

8–10 ounces (227–284 g) apple cider vinegar

Yield: 10 ounces

To make:

1. Place all the fresh herbs in a 12 ounce (340 gram) jar. Completely cover with vinegar.

2. Cover the jar and let sit in a warm spot for 4 weeks, shaking occasionally.

3. Strain the liquid.

4. If desired, combine with floral water of your choice.

QUEEN OF HUNGARY WATER BLENDS

To make a superior astringent, combine Queen of Hungary Water with a floral water that fits your skin type or individual preference (see previous recipe). Following are the recommended blending proportions:

Dry skin: 1 part Queen of Hungary Water to 4 parts floral water

Normal skin: 1 part Queen of Hungary Water to 2 parts floral water

Oily skin: 1 part Queen of Hungary Water to 1 part floral water

BAY RUM AFTERSHAVE

Next time you're in California, you have to make this tonic for the man in your life. But don't let him keep it all to himself; it is also a nice toner for women who like spicy scents. This recipe was inspired by the bay rum products offered in many mail-order catalogs.

2 cups (500 ml) fresh bay leaves

1 tablespoon (15 ml) dried, whole cloves

1 teaspoon (5 ml) ground ginger

1 teaspoon (5 ml) allspice

1 teaspoon (5 ml) fennel

2 cups (500 ml) rum

Yield: 2 cups (500 ml)

To make:

1. Fill a widemouthed jar with bay leaves, cloves, ginger, allspice, and fennel.

2. Cover the herbs with rum.

3. Let sit for 4 weeks in a warm place, shaking occasionally.

4. Strain out the herbs and rebottle the herbal liquid.

To use:

1. Dilute with orange blossom floral water (see box on page 101 for proportions).

2. Men should pour approximately 2 tablespoons in their hands, then splash on the face after shaving. Women, you'll feel refreshed splashing some on after washing up.

BLEMISH LINIMENT

Use this ointment on boils, acne, infected wounds, cuts, poison oak, and poison ivy. This recipe is my variation of Jethro Kloss' liniment (see *Back to Eden* for the original).

1 tablespoon (15 ml) dried goldenseal powder

2 tablespoons (30 ml) dried echinacea powder

2 tablespoons (30 ml) dried myrrh powder

2 teaspoons (10 ml) dried cayenne powder

2 cups (500 ml) 100-proof vodka

2 cups (500 ml) distilled water

Yield: 4 cups

To make:

1. Place herbs in a jar and cover with vodka.

2. Shake daily for 4 weeks.

3. Strain and rebottle the liquid, using 1 part liquid to 1 part distilled water.

To use:

1. Dab liniment onto a cotton ball.

2. Lightly rub on affected areas. If it is too harsh, dilute 1:2 instead (1 part liniment to 2 parts distilled water).

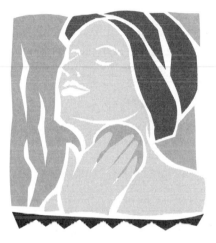

Herbal
Massage

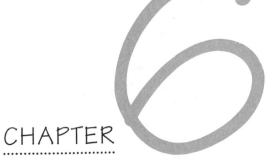

CHAPTER

Touch is an important component of good health. We all need to be touched. Many health practitioners now recommend at least one massage per month. Just think of what it would be like on planet Earth if everyone received a massage each month. I think it would be transformational. Unfortunately, though, some of us may have been touched inappropriately as children so that as adults we find it hard to trust others enough to let them touch us. Perhaps equally tragic are the children who were never touched as babies, and grow up unable to receive loving touch.

Please do lovingly touch your children and if you relate to any of the above, get the help you need to heal your past. We all deserve and need to be touched regularly.

TYPES OF MASSAGE

There are a variety of massage practices, but they may not all be styles that you enjoy. How do you choose the massage that is right for you? I think one of the easiest ways to end up happy with the massage you select is to evaluate yourself on a masculinity/femininity scale.

The more feminine, or yin, you are, the gentler your massage should be. The more masculine, or yang, you are, the more you'll appreciate a deeper, more vigorous massage. This is true for both men and women, because both men and women have yin and yang aspects to their being. I think of myself as leaning toward the feminine, and I hate a vigorous massage. It hurts me. My husband likes the opposite. One problem is that most of us give someone the type of massage we like to receive. Don't hesitate to tell your masseuse what you like, and to remind her as often as you need to. It's important that you receive the kind of massage you will enjoy most.

There are many different techniques and styles of massage. For more information, consult the bibliography (see page 92) or look for a mini-course on massage at your local adult education center. It's worth exploring all the options.

This chapter offers many easy formulas for creating oils that can be used with different massage techniques: herbal infused oils, aromatherapy oils, and a combination of the two.

A cream lotion and a moisturizing cream recipe are also included if you want to get a little fancier. The budget-conscious consumer can save a bundle by making her own blended herbal oils.

MASSAGE OILS AND LOTIONS

Massage often is done with straight vegetable oil. That's fine, especially for you minimalists out there. The next step up are aromatherapy oils, which are easy to make and offer the healing elements of both the herbs and their aroma. Herbal infused oils are a bit more work, but they offer the healing elements of the herbs you choose to infuse. You can also create a product with both if you want to get really fancy: Infuse the oil with herbs, then scent with a complementary essential oil.

Care and Storage of Oils

Oils are delicate. Light and heat destabilize them; protect your oils from both. Destabilized oils become rancid. Rancid oils are linked to cancer, so it is important to heed safeguards in making, using, and storing products with oils. Dark amber and cobalt blue bottles afford the most protection from light.

Unfortunately, even the oils purchased at health food stores are rarely packaged in dark containers, with the exception of olive oil, which is the least light sensitive. If you can, purchase oils in bulk from a supplier who has them in a dark container. If you've purchased oil in a clear glass container, either transfer it to a darker bottle or tape brown paper around the glass.

People who live in hot climates may need to refrigerate oil products for most of the year. Those in cooler climates may be

WHY USE NATURAL OILS?

Synthetic oils, petroleum products, and mineral oils create a barrier on the skin. This may seem helpful, but they do not allow the skin to breathe. Vegetable oils are closer to natural human oils and are better for people. Use the petroleum products on your car! Unfortunately, most commercial cosmetics contain mineral or synthetic oils. And if you go for a massage, a budget-conscious masseuse may also be using these products. Ask for a natural vegetable oil. And certainly do not skimp at home, either. (Familiarize yourself with the oils listed on pages 35–38.)

able to get away with storing them in a cool, dark basement. Make small quantities, and refrigerate products that you have heated to make if you are not using them daily.

Aromatherapy Scented Oils

Use pure essential oils rather than synthetic fragrance oils: That way you'll get the full therapeutic value of the scent. Choose the oils that call to you. I don't like to make things too fussy, so I usually choose the simplest method: one scent combined with one main oil, an antioxidant oil, and a few drops of vitamin E oil. But please don't let me stifle your imagination if you want to create blends. Blends are usually made with a top-note essential oil, a middle note, and a base note (see bibliography for books on aromatherapy).

SIMPLE LAVENDER OIL

⅔ cup (150 ml) grape-
    seed oil
⅓ cup (75 ml) wheat
    germ oil
10 drops vitamin E oil
6 drops lavender
    essential oil

Yield: 8 ounces

To make:
1. Pour all ingredients into a dark bottle that has a spout.
2. Shake well.
To use:
1. Shake well before each use.
2. Pour the oil into your hands to warm before putting it on the body.
3. Massage into your body using a circular motion.

RED ROSE OIL

⅔ cup (150 ml) grape-
seed oil
1 teaspoon (5 ml)
alkanet root
⅓ cup (75 ml) wheat
germ oil
10 drops vitamin E oil
6 drops rose essen-
tial oil

Yield: 8 ounces

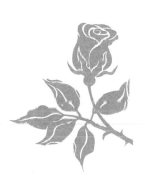

To make:
1. Pour the grapeseed oil and the alkanet
root into the top of a double boiler.
2. Gently heat the water bath of the double
boiler on the lowest heat.
3. Once the desired degree of redness is
achieved in the oil, remove from heat and
strain out the alkanet.
4. Add the wheat germ oil, vitamin E, and
essential oil to the red oil.
5. Pour all ingredients into a dark bottle that
has a spout.
6. Shake well.
To use:
1. Shake well before each use.
2. Pour the oil into your hands to warm
before putting it on the body.
3. Massage into your body using a circular
motion.

Herbal Infused Oils

To make essential oils and expeller pressed oils, special equipment and often large quantities of herbs or flowers are needed.
Do you want to harness the healing power of herbs and flowers
in a vegetable oil base for only a fraction of the price of commercial herb and flower oils? Good news! You can make your
own infused oils. See recipe on page 178 that can be used to
relieve nerve damage and muscle pain. Substitute 2 cups olive
oil for sesame/olive oil combination, if desired.

CREAMY LOTION

This wonderful lotion is my adaptation of a Rosemary Gladstar recipe.

2 tablespoons (30 ml) fresh chamomile flowers

2 tablespoons (30 ml) fresh rose buds

2 tablespoons (30 ml) fresh comfrey

2 tablespoons (30 ml) fresh lavender

2 tablespoons (30 ml) fresh calendula

2 fresh sage leaves

1 sprig fresh rosemary

2 tablespoons (30 ml) dried witch hazel bark

2 tablespoons (30 ml) fresh lemon balm

1¼ cups (300 ml) apricot kernel, almond, or grapeseed oil

¼ cup (50 ml) cocoa butter

⅔ cup (150 ml) coconut oil

5 drops essential oil (optional)

1 sterilized, 12-ounce (340-gram) wide-mouthed jar

Yield: Approximately 12 ounces (340 g)

To make:

1. Harvest fresh herbs in midmorning, if possible.

2. Place herbs on paper towels and allow to wilt overnight.

3. Fill jar with wilted herbs.

4. Completely cover the herbs with apricot, almond, or grapeseed oil.

5. Each day for the next week, poke herbs down into the oil to release any captured gases. For the three following weeks, do this once a week.

6. After 4 weeks, strain the herbs from the oil.

7. To the infused oil, add cocoa butter and coconut oil. Warm until all ingredients melt together. Scent with the essential oil of your choice.

To use:

1. Pour oil into the palm of your hands to warm.

2. Gently massage into the skin.

MOISTURING CREAM MASSAGE

If you prefer to use a moisturizing cream for massage, see the recipes for Rose Pink Face Moisurizer, Lavender Blue Face Moisturizer, and Orange Blossom Face Cream found on pages 96–98.

BASIC MASSAGE STROKES FOR REVITALIZATION

There are many different types of massage and therapeutic touch, and plenty of good books on the subject (see bibliography). Here I offer a simple explanation of a few beginning strokes you can do at home that are quite beneficial.

EFFLEURAGE

This is a gliding stroke over the surface of the skin, usually done with oil or a massage cream. Massage normally starts with light effleurage to gently connect with the person, soothing their nervous system. Gradually, deeper strokes with more pressure may be applied to increase the circulation of blood and lymph.

PETRISSAGE

This kneading movement lifts, presses, and rolls muscle tissue away from the bone to increase circulation of blood and lymph and to detoxify the muscles.

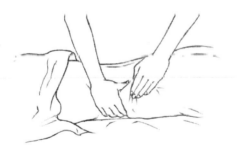

BEGIN WITH GENTLE STROKES

I do not believe in "no pain, no gain." While some sports massage therapists might argue for deep and penetrating massage, rubbing, or scrubbing, I think it is always best to start out gently. A light massage can be quite helpful. It also gives you a chance to identify sensitive areas and pressure preferences, whether you are applying the massage to yourself or to someone else. I urge you to use gentle and loving touch. It makes a big difference. And do ask to be told if you are hurting your "client."

COMPRESSION

Compression is direct pressure to the body and affects muscular, nervous, and energy systems. This technique is done with the thumbs, the whole hand, and even the elbows.

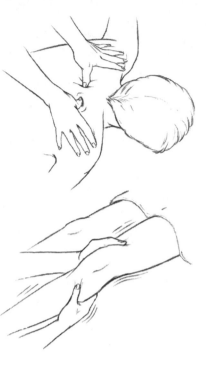

ROCKING

Rocking is a smooth, rhythmic motion that soothes the nervous system. Gently shaking the limbs or rocking parts of the torso encourages the receiver to let go of tension.

DOING MASSAGE AT HOME

In doing massage at home, it is assumed that you have a relationship with the individual you are touching. Most states require a license for massages done for pay. You should be aware of any health conditions of the person you are working on; ask the person if you are not. It can be quite helpful, especially for repeat treatments, to note where a person experiences pain or blockages. Monthly massage can help to alleviate pain and improve circulation.

Getting Ready

Preparation is essential in creating a quality massage experience. Select a place of solitude where you won't be interrupted. A massage table adjusted for your height is ideal, but cushioning a long table or even using a bed or sofa can also be effective. Set up the table so that you can get around all sides, if possible. Make up the table or bed with both a bottom and a top sheet.

Another important factor is warmth. Warmth helps the muscles relax and is essential to a good massage. When lying in the prone position, the body tends to lose heat. Oil on the skin results in it becoming easily chilled. Make sure the room is warm when you start; bring in a space heater if necessary. Also use blankets as needed. Select music that is soothing and pleasing to your "client."

STEP-BY-STEP MASSAGE

This is a simple technique. You may want to learn other massage techniques through your local adult education center. Better yet, take the course with your partner.

- Top and bottom sheets
- Pillow
- Blanket or two
- Massage lotion, oil, or cream
- Bowl
- Relaxing music
- Space heater

1. Wash your hands thoroughly before the massage and trim fingernails if necessary.
2. Pour 4 ounces (100 g) of oil into the bowl to start for easy access.
3. Oil your hands and rub them together to warm the oil.
4. Start with your "client" lying face up with his or her body covered by a sheet (and blanket, if needed). Apply the oil to the throat using gentle side-to-side strokes (see page 87 for illustration of facial strokes).
5. Gently swipe across the chin, above the lips, and then across the forehead.
6. Using the fingertips, gently massage in upward strokes, starting at the jaw outside the mouth, coming up along the side of the nose, then across the bridge of the nose.
7. Make several spiraling, circular motions spanning the entire forehead, ending up above and outside the eyes.
8. Press the cheekbones using slight pressure from the outside to inside.
9. Use a spiral, circular stroke on the cheeks.

10. Press along the sides of the neck, working outward to the shoulders.

11. Massage the crown of the head using the fingertips. Press gently, working down and around to the back of the skull.

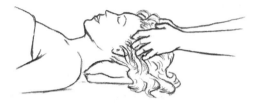

12. Uncover one arm, leaving the rest of the body draped. Gently holding the wrist, shake the arm from side to side. With both hands around the arm, gently squeeze, working back and forth starting at the shoulder and working down to the hand.

13. Do the same on the other arm and then each leg.

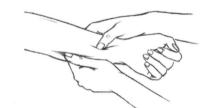

14. Have the "client" turn over, and work on the back. Starting at the base of the spine, gently push on the spine, working up to the top of the shoulders. Rub the shoulders and top of the back all over.

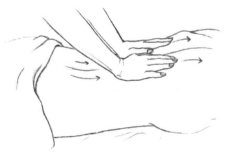

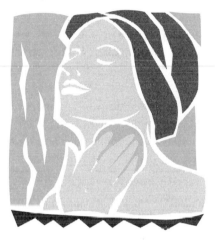

Herbal Body Wraps and Skin Treatments

CHAPTER 7

Body wraps and herbal skin treatments are designed to increase circulation, remove toxins, and promote smooth, soft, supple skin. The skin is the body's largest organ of elimination. Good circulation to the skin helps rid the body of harmful substances and enhances secretion of natural oils, which moisturize the skin and keep the body healthy. Blood flowing to the skin brings oxygen to the surface; blood and lymph flowing away from the skin release and eliminate toxins. By stimulating circulation, the body is better able to eliminate impurities.

Over the centuries, various cultures have developed techniques to enhance circulation and produce healthy, glowing skin. Most of these involve creating friction on the skin, or exfoliating, a process that assists the blood and lymph systems in releasing wastes. The Hindu tradition of Ayurvedic healing uses a silk-mitt exfoliation technique. Romans used dry brushing. Mexican and surrounding Central American cultures weave agate fibers into washcloths or pads to rub the skin while bathing. All the seafaring cultures have traditionally used sea salt, seaweed, and the sun for increasing circulation. (Century plant, or agave, is woven to form ayate products.)

Many of these time-tested techniques are featured at today's most elegant spas. In this chapter, you will learn how you can practice them at home. I also show you how you can prepare and apply luxurious herb, fruit, and vegetable body scrubs, wraps, and masks, along with thalassotherapy, to create pampering and nurturing sessions at your own home spa.

CAUTION

The treatments presented in this chapter are beneficial for addressing a wide range of health concerns. However, you should consult your doctor before engaging in the treatments, especially if you have varicose veins or circulation or heart problems.

THE BENEFITS OF INCREASED CIRCULATION

Most of us have sluggish skin and don't realize it. You may have heard the saying, "Animals sweat, men perspire, and women merely glow." In truth, it would be better if we were more like animals on this account. The inability to sweat all over, especially when exercising or in a sauna, is a symptom of poor skin elimination due to poor circulation. Dull complexion, cold hands and feet, and constipation are other signs of poor circulation. The treatments in this chapter alleviate these conditions by increasing circulation, bringing warmth to the extremities, improving the complexion, and acting as a mild laxative. Thus, no need to feel that you're being overindulgent with these treatments — they are part of staying healthy and feeling well!

Weight Control and Cellulite

Unwelcome weight gain and cellulite can also often be managed by increasing blood circulation to the skin on a daily basis. Good circulation is not just a surface phenomenon; it makes for healthier internal organs as well. Healthy organ functioning aids metabolism and weight management.

Weight gain sometimes can be remedied or controlled by raising your activity level, which in turn increases circulation. The sluggishness of weight gain may show up in the skin as dullness or pallor. Increasing circulation helps let go of the pounds and in turn creates more vibrant, alive skin — and the healthy glow that goes along with it.

DANGERS OF OVERUSING SOAP AND MOISTURIZERS

Two everyday hygiene practices that inhibit circulation and block the skin surface are excessive use of soap and overuse of moisturizing creams, especially those containing petroleum products. While Americans are often surprised at the European practice of bathing less frequently, we are actually the ones who are caught up in a "hygiene paranoia." Manufacturers of hygiene products play on these fears of being "stinky" or in some way unattractive with the heavy emphasis on deodorizing in their advertisements.

Regardless, our practice of washing all of our body with soap is unnecessary

MINIMIZE USE OF MOISTURIZING CREAM

Body moisturizing creams should be applied lightly and sparingly. By increasing the use of the circulation-enhancing techniques suggested in this chapter, you can gradually diminish your dependence on moisture creams. As a result of exfoliation, the natural oils in your skin will come to the surface to create a baby-bottom softness without any added cream.

and can even be detrimental to good circulation, not to mention costly. Don't fret if you love good soaps; they certainly have their place. Soaps are meant for the hairy parts of the body, that is, the hair, underarms, and pubic region. Soaps are okay for sweaty and dirty areas as well, such as under the breasts, your hands and feet, or other parts that may get dirty as a result of your daily work. Other parts of your body, however, even if you are a man with a lot of hair on your back, are best washed simply with water or possibly a slightly acid rinse of water and vinegar or lemon juice.

The natural pH of the skin is slightly acidic. By constantly putting basic (as opposed to acidic) products such as soap on the skin, it is constantly fighting to get back to its natural pH. The result is dry, itchy skin, and the need for moisture creams.

Moisture creams, unfortunately, also inhibit the skin's natural functions. Most of the commercial products available contain petroleum-based ingredients that block the natural breathing of the skin and inhibit circulation. Creams with purer ingredients, however, may be very expensive. You can save both your money and your skin by making your own moisture creams. The recipes in chapter 5 (see pages 96–98) for the face and neck are inexpensive enough to use all over your body.

A WARNING FOR ITCHY-SKIN SUFFERERS

If you have itchy skin, be especially careful to avoid using soap excessively, bathing in a tub full of soapsuds, and over-moisturizing your skin. All of these practices interfere with your skin's ability to maintain its natural pH. Your itching may clear up by omitting soap or by bathing in or rinsing with a combination of water and vinegar or lemon juice.

EXFOLIATION TECHNIQUES

Exfoliating the skin is a process by which you use an abrasive surface to rub the skin (usually before showering), scraping away any dead cells on your skin's surface, increasing circulation, and making the skin glow. If you have delicate skin, please don't give up on exfoliation. Start out gently and in no time you'll be able to tolerate more vigorous scrubs and rubs. Don't be alarmed if you start to notice a few blemishes; this is normal as the skin starts to slough off impurities, and it will diminish as your skin gets healthier.

LOOFAH SPONGE RUB

You will find a variety of loofah products in the health and beauty aisle of many drugstores. Experiment with using whole loofahs, sewing a piece into a washcloth to create a mitt, or making a disk of the softer part for your face.

Materials needed: Loofah sponge, style of your choice.
To use: Wet the loofah in the shower and rub it all over your body to invigorate the skin. You can also use it to slough off dry skin before showering. Standing in the tub, rub the loofah over your dry body in a circular motion, starting at the extremities and working toward the torso.

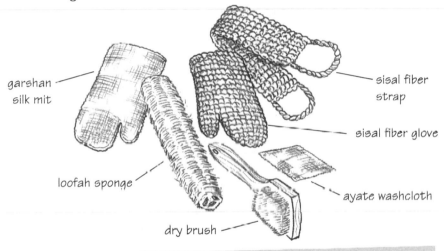

garshan silk mit

loofah sponge

dry brush

sisal fiber strap

sisal fiber glove

ayate washcloth

GROWING LOOFAH

The loofah sponge is not a sponge at all — it's a plant (part of the cucumber family) that you can grow in your garden. You may be able to obtain seeds from a purchased loofah; shake it and see if any fall out. If not, you can purchase loofah seeds at most garden centers. The seeds are slow to germinate, so start them indoors and transplant them out later. The plants enjoy growing on a trellis for support and take about 75 days to produce gourds. When the skin turns brown, it is time to harvest. Dry the gourds, then soak them in water until the outer skin disappears, and you've got your exfoliating sponge. These make great gifts, too.

ROMAN DRY BRUSHING

The stiffer the bristles on your brush, the better the lymphatic stimulation you'll generate. If you have trouble finding a dry brush at your local natural food or health store, see the resource list on page 190.

Materials needed: Natural bristle brush (palm-size; also available with optional stick for use on back).

To use: Standing in the bathtub (to catch the falling skin), brush the dry skin all over your body, starting with the fingertips and arms and working inward toward the torso. Next, brush your legs and move upward toward the torso. Some areas may be more sensitive than others, for instance, the breasts and neck, yet the treatment is quite good for them as well. The more often you do this treatment, the less sensitive your skin will become. Once or twice a day is recommended.

RECOMMENDED EXFOLIATING TECHNIQUES

It's important to brush or rub your body in the particular sequence that is most conducive to circulation. Begin by rubbing the extremities (arms and legs) and working inward to the torso. This encourages the blood flow in toward the heart. Then, rub your torso to encourage the blood to flow out from the heart through the organs and to the entire body.

These exfoliation techniques can be used on all parts of the body except the face. Gradually, as you use these techniques more and more, you will find that your skin tolerates a more vigorous scrub or rub. But be careful not to get carried away and rub or brush your skin to the point of bleeding. If you are like me and tend to have itchy skin, the brushing and rubbing may feel so good that you overdo it. One way to treat the itchiness is to take regular vinegar baths (see page 140).

GARSHAN SILK-MITT TREATMENT

This exfoliation technique comes from the Ayurvedic healing techniques developed in India to create vigor, energy, and balance in the body, mind, emotions, and beyond. If you know someone with rough hands you won't need the mitt — just talk that person into giving you a rub with his or her bare hands.

Materials needed: ¼ yard (23 cm) raw silk, needle and thread (or sewing machine). Makes 1 mitt.

To make: Cut two mitten-shaped pieces from the raw silk, using the pattern in the appendix (page 194). With right sides together, sew a ⅝" seam around the mitt, leaving the bottom open. Turn the mitt right side out.

To use: With the mitt on your hand, scrub your entire body, wet or dry, starting from the extremities and moving inward toward the torso. This is good preparation for the cellulite body wrap (see page 128).

AYATE FIBER CLOTH RUB

The century plant grows in the Southwest and Mexico and has been used for centuries by Native peoples for exfoliating. Look for products made from ayate or agave in a health food store. The loosely woven cloth shrinks to a finer weave when put in water.

To use: Wet the ayate cloth and rub it over your entire body when taking a shower or bath, starting from the extremities and moving inward to the torso.

SISAL FIBER RUB

Similar to the ayate fiber cloth, sisal fiber cloth is often made into gloves and back straps for rubbing on the body. Look for these products in your local health food store (or see resource list).

To use: Wet the sisal fiber glove or strap and rub over entire body when showering or bathing, working from the extremities inward. The glove is especially good for rubbing on fleshy areas such as the thighs.

HERBAL BODY SCRUBS

Another way to exfoliate the skin and remove toxins is to make a grainy herbal body scrub. Any number of fruits, grains, herbs, minerals, and vegetables can been used alone or in combination to make scrubs. Most substances that are safe to eat are also safe to use on the skin, provided you do not have an allergy. Several recipes for herbal body scrubs follow, but please don't limit yourself to these combinations. You can really let your imagination run wild: Mix up your own concoctions, based on the ingredients you happen to have on hand or your favorite fruits, herbs, and vegetables. When you're experimenting, try making small batches before you go to full-scale production.

AVOCADO MOISTURE SCRUB

Tired of sprouting or just throwing away avocado pits? Here's a great way to use them, and it gives you low-fat dieters an excuse to splurge. Avocado, high in fat and oil, is very therapeutic for dry skin.

2–3 fresh avocado pits
1 cup (250 ml) milk, water, or yogurt

Yield: 1 treatment

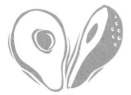

To make:
1. Let the avocado pits dry for a few days, but not to the point of becoming rock hard (or they will break your spice mill).
2. Using a spice mill or coffee grinder, grind the dried avocado pits to create a grainy, mealy powder.
3. Add the water, milk, or yogurt to the powder and mix to form a paste.

To use:
1. Sitting or standing in the bathtub or shower, pat avocado paste all over your body using a circular motion. Start from the tips of the extremities and work toward the torso. Don't forget to apply this mixture to your face, too.
2. Leave on for 10 minutes, then shower, first with warm water, then cooler water.
3. Pat dry.

OATMEAL ALMOND BODY SCRUB

Many ground nuts make excellent scrubs: With their high fat content, they moisturize while exfoliating. Oatmeal is quite moisturizing, making this recipe especially good for dry or itchy skin. Be sure to tie up your hair or wear a shower cap, as this can get messy.

1 cup (250 ml) oatmeal
1 cup (250 ml) white cosmetic clay
½ cup (125 ml) almonds
½ cup (125 ml) dried rose petals
½ cup (125 ml) dried lemon balm
½ cup (125 ml) yogurt
Juice of 1 lemon

Yield: 1 treatment

To make:
1. Grind or powder the oatmeal, almonds, rose petals, and lemon balm separately using a spice mill or blender, leaving some grit in each.
2. In a large bowl, mix all the dry ingredients with a wire whisk.
3. Add the lemon juice and yogurt and blend thoroughly.
4. Add water as needed.

To use:
1. Sitting in the bathtub, slather on the scrub. Using a circular motion, start with the toes and work up the leg.
2. Next work on the arms, starting with the hands and working toward the torso.
3. Using a circular motion, massage in the mix to the torso.
4. Sit in the tub for 10 minutes, allowing the clay mix to dry on the skin.
5. Shower or bathe in warm water, gently rinsing the skin.
6. Pat dry.

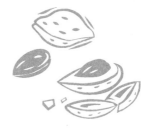

HERBAL BODY MASKS AND POLISHES

Body masks, designed to moisturize the skin, use ingredients with emollient, humectant, nourishing, and healing properties. As with the body scrubs, the masks use the fleshier parts of fruits, herbs, vegetables, dairy products, and oils. These treatments are similar to those offered in some of the more fabulous spas. Don't be afraid to use these as a springboard for developing your own personalized recipes.

APPLE PULP POMADE

Especially good for those with sensitive skin, this recipe is great to make at the height of apple season.

15 medium-size apples (McIntosh work well)
½ cup (125 ml) apricot kernel oil
1 tablespoon (15 ml) Zest of lemon

Yield: 1 treatment

To make:
1. Cut up apples and put in a large pot.
2. Add a little water, as needed.
3. Simmer and mash till the mixture is the consistency of applesauce, approximately 30 minutes.
4. Pour off excess water.
5. Add apricot kernel oil and lemon zest; mix well. Use while still warm.

To use:
1. While sitting in the tub or shower, slather the warm apple mixture all over your body, and hair, too, if you like.
2. Rest in the tub with the mixture on for 10 minutes.
3. Shower in warm water.
4. Pat dry.

CUCUMBER BODY PIZZA

Don't have the time or the inclination for mixing lotions and potions today? Are you suffering from the "itches" or poison ivy? Try this Cucumber Body Pizza. It is cooling, draws out the itch, and isn't messy. You may want to have a partner around to apply the cucumber slices for you.

3–5 cucumbers

Yield: 1 treatment

To make:
1. Thinly slice the cucumbers and place on a plate.
To use:
1. Lie face down in a comfortable position in a warm place. Have a friend place cucumber slices all over the back side of your body, so they are just touching but not overlapping. Use about half the total slices.
2. Rest quietly for 10 to 20 minutes to allow the cucumber slices and juice to penetrate your skin.
3. Remove the slices.
4. Turn over and apply the rest of the slices to your front side. Relax for 10 to 20 minutes. You may want to shower afterwards, but it is best not to for at least 4 hours, as the cucumber will continue to work on the skin during that time

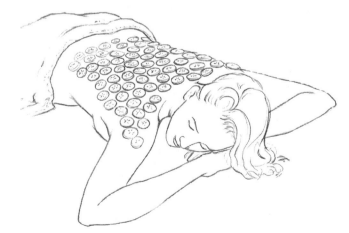

SALT GLOW

The Salt Glow is a vigorous circulatory stimulant that removes dead surface cells and dirt, leaving your skin soft and gleaming. Salt Glow stimulates the secretion of your natural skin oils and is especially helpful for sluggish skin. You may fear being dried out with this rub, but I find my moderately dry skin loves this treatment, and leaves me feeling like a baby's bottom all over. The salts encourage the skin to secrete its natural oils.

2 cups (500 ml) coarse sea salt
¼ cup (50 ml) water

Yield: 1 treatment

To use:
1. Place the salt in a bowl and wet it with the water.
2. Fill the tub ankle-deep with warm water and step into the tub.
3. Starting with your arms, wet them and then rub the salt vigorously on the skin, moving from the fingertips to shoulders until the skin is aglow.
4. Next wet your legs. Now rub on the salt, beginning at your feet and moving up to your thighs.
5. Next, wet the torso and then rub on the salt in a circular motion.
6. Once your whole body has been rubbed, sit in the warm tub of water to relax, allowing the salt to work on your skin while sitting in the ankle-deep water for a few minutes.
7. Rinse with warm water and follow with a cool rinse.

Variations:
◆ Substitute ½ cup (125 ml) grapeseed oil (or almond, apricot kernel, or olive oil) for the ¼ cup (50 ml) water.
◆ Add 6 to 8 drops of essential oil to the straight salt or salt and oil mix.

CAUTION

Avoid applying salt on the face or on any cuts or broken skin.

AROMATHERAPY BATH SALTS

Each pure essential oil has a scent and character all its own. Select one for your Salt Glow that has the therapeutic benefits to suit your needs and mood. Here are a few of the more common ones you might want to try, along with their benefits. For more information about aromatherapy, consult Colleen K. Dodt's *The Essential Oils Book* (see bibliography).

- ◆ **Chamomile:** relaxing and calming
- ◆ **Clary Sage:** warming; promotes feelings of well-being
- ◆ **Basil:** relieves mental fatigue and nervousness
- ◆ **Eucalyptus:** promotes clear breathing
- ◆ **Jasmine:** antidepressant; supports feelings of confidence
- ◆ **Lavender:** soothing
- ◆ **Orange:** cheering
- ◆ **Peppermint:** stimulating, increases energy
- ◆ **Pine:** alleviates fatigue

PUMPKIN SLATHER

Like so many of the squash vegetables, pumpkins are excellent moisturizers for your body.

1 small pumpkin
1 cup (250 ml) yogurt
Juice from 1 lemon

Yield: 1 treatment

To make:

1. Cut up the pumpkin, removing skin and scooping out pulp. Place the flesh in a pot with a small amount of water.

2. Cook the pumpkin until mashable with a potato masher.

3. Remove from heat, mash pumpkin, and add yogurt and lemon juice. Use while still warm.

To use:

1. Sit in the tub or shower, and slather the warm pumpkin mixture all over your dry body, and hair, too, if you like.

2. Rest in the tub with the mixture on your body for 10 minutes.

3. Shower in warm water.

4. Pat dry.

HERBAL BODY WRAPS

In spas the world over, clients pay big bucks for these treatments. Wraps are credited with creating all kinds of miracles, including weight loss and cellulite removal. Regardless of whether these claims are true, this is a great way to be pampered. You may need to recruit assistance with the wrapping part of this treatment. What a great Valentine's Day ritual for you to share with a partner.

BASIC HERBAL WRAP FORMULA

2 cups (500 ml) fresh herbs (1 cup [250 ml] dried)

1 large cotton sheet ripped into 2-inch-wide (5-cm) strips, each as long as possible

Clean plastic drop cloth or tarp

Large basin or spaghetti pot

Yield: 1 treatment

To make:
1. Place the herbs in the basin or pot.
2. Pour boiling water over the herbs and cover. Let steep for 5 minutes.
3. Remove as many herbs as you can from the pot using a strainer.
4. Add the sheet strips to the pot and steep for 5 more minutes.

To use:
1. Exfoliate using your preferred method, then shower before using this treatment.
2. Lay the drop cloth or tarp on a comfortable recliner, chair, or bed — preferably in a warm room.

SUGGESTED HERBS FOR USE IN A BODY WRAP

For stimulation and energy: peppermint, rosemary, juniper, lemon peel
For relaxation: lavender, clary sage, chamomile, tangerine peel
For healing and antiseptic properties: calendula, eucalyptus, tea tree, lavender
For aches and pains: 1 cup (250 ml) Epsom salts plus rosemary, lavender, or eucalyptus
For itchy skin: red clover plus 1 cup (250 ml) apple cider vinegar or lemon juice

3. Remove the sheet strips one by one, wringing out the liquid. Wrap each strip around your body snugly. Start with the arms, then follow with the legs, the torso, and the head.

4. Once all the strips are wrapped and the body is covered, sit in the chair and wrap the drop cloth or tarp around your body.

5. Cover yourself with a few blankets and relax quietly for 10 minutes.

6. Unwrap the strips from your body and slowly emerge from your cocoon.

7. It is best not to shower for at least 4 hours afterwards and preferably not for 24 hours.

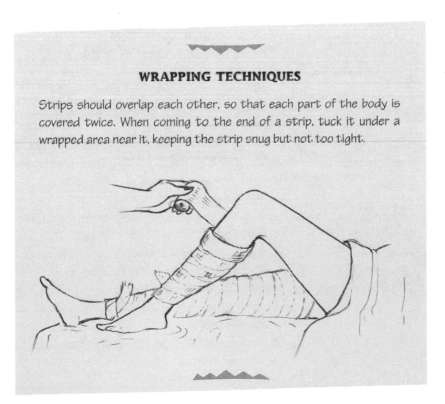

WRAPPING TECHNIQUES

Strips should overlap each other, so that each part of the body is covered twice. When coming to the end of a strip, tuck it under a wrapped area near it, keeping the strip snug but not too tight.

CELLULITE BODY WRAP

This body wrap is aimed at reducing those little cottage cheese bumps that occur on many women's derrieres and thighs. It is most effective when done in a warm room. You may need to enlist some help with wrapping the cellophane.

8 drops of grapefruit essential oil
2 drops each of essential oils of thyme, fennel, lavender, geranium, juniper berry
2 cups (500 ml) almond oil
Cellophane wrap

Yield: 1 treatment

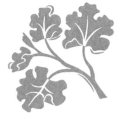

To use:

1. Turn up the heat in the bathroom or bedroom.

2. In a plastic squirt bottle, combine the essential oils with the almond oil, shaking well.

3. Exfoliate the skin using your preferred method (loofah, silk mitt, dry brush, or ayate or sisal fiber — see pages 116–119).

4. While standing in the shower or bathtub or on a towel in your bedroom, knead the oil mixture generously into the skin on your arms, legs, and torso, avoiding the face and neck.

5. Encase your legs in cellophane beginning at the toes and working up to the thighs. I have found it easier to apply the cellophane when the whole cellophane roll is cut in half or thirds to 2-inch (5-cm) widths. Wrap snugly, but don't cut off the circulation.

6. Wrap your arms, beginning at the hands and moving up to the upper arms. Complete by wrapping the torso.

7. Relax in a warm room for 20 minutes. You can make the tub as comfy as possible with a pillow for your head, or sit on a comfortable chair or bed that you've covered with a towel.

8. Remove the cellophane wrap from your body; shower first with warm water, then with cooler water.

9. Pat skin dry.

BASIC CLAY BODY WRAP FORMULA

Use this French clay body wrap at least once a month to remove toxins from the body and leave the skin soft and smooth.

½ cup (125 ml) dried herbs

1 cup (250 ml) distilled water

1 cup (250 ml) French, green, or red clay

1 tablespoon (15 ml) almond or apricot kernel oil

1 tablespoon (15 ml) yogurt

3 drops essential oil of your choice

2 large bedsheets torn into 6-inch-wide (15-cm) strips, each as long as possible

1 large pot of boiling water

New medium-size paintbrush

Yield: 1 treatment

To make:

1. Place the herbs in a clean, 10-ounce (284-gram) glass jar.

2. Bring the distilled water to a boil.

3. Pour the boiling water over the herbs, cover, and allow to steep for 10 minutes to make an herbal infusion.

4. Put the clay in a medium-size bowl; add the almond or apricot kernel oil and yogurt and mix.

5. Add the herbal infusion to the clay mixture, herbs and all.

6. Add the bedsheet strips to the large pot of boiling water.

To use:

1. Bring the clay mixture and the pot with strips to the bathroom.

2. Standing in the bathtub, begin applying the clay mixture to your legs with the paintbrush, starting at the toes and working up to the thighs.

3. Wring out one of the fabric strips and begin wrapping your legs from the toes up. Continue to wrap snugly (but not cutting off the circulation), using more strips as needed.

4. Repeat step 3 for your arms, starting with the fingertips and working up to the shoulders.

5. Apply clay to torso and wrap, as in step 3.

6. Relax in the tub for 10 to 20 minutes.

7. Unwrap your body and shower with tepid water.

8. Pat dry.

HOT AND COLD STIMULATION

You may know about the Scandinavian practice of sitting in a warm sauna and then going out to jump in the snow. This combination of hot and cold body immersions is good for the circulation and is a great way to stay warm in winter. Most people cringe at the suggestion of taking a cold-water shower, especially in winter. But listen up, all you undershirt, turtleneck, and sweater people who are cold all winter: This is your cure.

Consider how chilled you usually feel when stepping out of a warm shower into the cooler air of your home. You can avoid this chilling sensation by showering first with warm water and then with cold water, which stimulates your circulation. After this shocking treatment, when you step out of the shower, your body responds immediately by bringing more blood to the surface and creating warmth, since the last sensation you felt in the shower was colder than the air outside it. Your body is warming up, rather than chilling down!

Hot and Cold Stimulating Shower

1. Shower as usual.

2. Before the shower is over, turn the water to the coldest temperature you can stand for 15 seconds, exposing all your body parts to the water, especially the nape of the neck.

3. Turn the water to the hottest you can stand for 15 seconds, again exposing all parts to the water. Note: Be sure you have a scald guard on your faucet, or that the temperature of the water does not exceed 110°F.

4. Turn the water back to the coldest you can tolerate for another 15 seconds. (Screaming and shouting are optional!)

5. Turn off the water. Towel dry, and notice how warm you feel.

THALASSOTHERAPY

Thalassotherapy is a Greek word used to refer to spa treatments that employ seawater and seaweed. Perhaps you think of salty seawater as drying, but these treatments are actually wonderful for dry skin and cellulite. Seaweed also increases circulation, thus helping to firm the skin and reduce fat accumulation.

SEAWEED BODY WRAP

You may need some help wrapping the gauze around your body for this treatment. When you're finished, the gauze can be rinsed and laundered and then used again.

2 cups (500 ml) clay of your choice
½ cup (125 ml) kelp powder
½ cup (125 ml) dulse powder
Juice from 1 lemon, divided in two
1 cup (250 ml) hot to warm water, divided in two
Enough gauze to cover your body
2 or 3 large beach towels

Yield: 1 treatment

To make:

1. In a large bowl, mix together the clay and seaweed powders with a wire whisk.

2. Place half the mixture in another bowl, then add the juice of ½ lemon and ½ cup hot to warm water, mixing to form a paste (reserve the rest of the lemon juice and water to add to the rest of the mixture when you need it).

To use:

1. Prepare your skin for the treatment first by dry brushing or exfoliating with another method of your choice (see pages 116–119).

2. Crank up the heat in the bathroom if possible, or bring in a space heater.

3. Standing in the bathtub or shower, first wet the skin. Then slather the seaweed mix onto your skin, starting with the feet.

4. Start wrapping the gauze firmly in an upward fashion around the clay-seaweed mixture on your body, beginning at the toes and working up the legs. Don't cut off the circulation, but keep it snug.

5. After both legs are covered, work from your fingers up your arms. When you run out of the mixture, add the juice and water to the other half of the recipe you had set aside.

6. Wrap the torso next, then the hair and neck, avoiding the face.

7. Lie back in the tub, covering yourself with beach towels, and get cozy for 20 minutes.

8. Remove the gauze from you body. Shower with warm water, then with cool water.

9. Pat dry.

THALASSOTHERAPY BODY MASK

This clay body mask helps remove toxins from the skin, leaving a healthy, glowing softness. This treatment is best done in a warm bathroom.

1 cup (250 ml) white cosmetic clay
½ cup (125 ml) kelp flakes or powder
½ cup (125 ml) dulse flakes
1 tablespoon (15 ml) sea salt
½ cup (125 ml) aloe vera gel
¼ cup (50 ml) water

Yield: 1 treatment

To make:
1. In a large bowl, mix together all the dry ingredients using a wire whisk.
2. Add the aloe vera gel and water to form a paste.

To use:
1. Standing in the bathtub, spread the paste all over your face and body, working from the tips of the extremities toward the torso.
2. Relax and allow the paste to dry for 20 minutes.
3. Shower off with warm water, rinsing thoroughly.

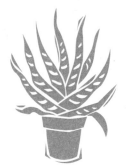

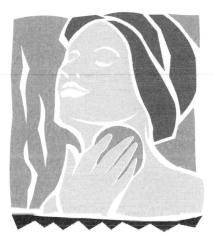

Herbal
Bathing
Rituals

CHAPTER

Bathing has long been a favored art for those who cannot resist the lure of calming, cleansing waters. These pleasure seekers are not new to our time but in fact are ancient. Early civilizations developed at the edges of rivers, lakes, and oceans, clearly recognizing the purifying, life-giving essence of water. The sacred use of water is central to many religions: Consider Christian baptism, Islamic preparation for prayer of ablutions, and the Native American sweat lodge, for example.

Bathing is still one of the most important rituals of our time. My bathroom is my sanctuary. I can't think of a more divine daily practice than bathing by candlelight. Water alone is quite pleasant, and being a purist and always looking for the least time-consuming preparations, I appreciate the uncomplicated in life. To enhance the sensory pleasure of the bathing experience, try some of the following simple, yet exotic, ideas. Bath products make wonderful gifts for yourself and for others. I include recipes for a variety of bath crystals, bath bubbles, milk baths, vinegar baths, and steam baths, along with information on how to use compresses and poultices and sitz baths for bathing and healing small areas of your body. (See chapter 9 for hand soaks and footbaths.)

SOAP

If you've ever made soap from scratch, you know it can be great fun but a little messy — and it may be more time-consuming than your schedule allows. (If you haven't tried making soap from scratch and are intrigued, I recommend Susan Miller Cavitch's *The Natural Soap Book* [see bibliography].)

GIFT IDEA

Lavender soap balls make lovely gifts. Place the soap balls in a soap dish and cover them with purple or lavender tulle. Tie with ribbon or raffia and a few sprigs of dried lavender. Several of my students who own bed-and-breakfasts have discovered how easy it is to create these special touches for their guests. But you don't have to wait to own a B&B; you can make them right now.

LAVENDER SOAP BALLS

This recipe enables you to create a beautiful product from simple ingredients in just a short time. This is a fun project to do with children, and it's especially good for those who have to be nagged to wash their hands!

2 bars mild, unscented soap (castile or vegetable-based)

½ cup (125 ml) dried lavender blossoms

5 drops essential oil of lavender

¼ cup (50 ml) warm water

Yield: Approximately 12 soap balls

To make:

1. Using a cheese grater, grate the soap bars into a large bowl.

2. Add the lavender blossoms to the grated soap.

3. Add the essential oil to the soap mixture, combining thoroughly.

4. Add the warm water and stir.

5. Roll heaping tablespoons of the mix into balls.

6. Place on a cookie sheet and allow to air-dry completely, which will take approximately 2 days.

BATH CRYSTALS

You'll find a variety of herbal and aromatherapy bath crystals at almost any pharmacy, health food emporium, or department store. I usually bring one or two of these prepackaged products to my classes to show students to demystify the "exotic" ingredients on the label. Desert salt sounds pretty extravagant, for instance. How can you obtain it short of taking a trip to the Sahara? How about a stroll down the laundry detergent aisle in your local supermarket? Yes, borax, the 20-mule-team stuff, is actually desert salt. Soda ash is another exotic name for a common household staple — baking soda. Since the beginning of time, individuals have used salts for skin treatments. None of these ingredients costs much. By making your own products you can save money, and at the same time customize the blend to fit your tastes and needs.

FINE CRYSTAL BATHING SAND

You'll see this product packaged in fancy jars or envelopes with a hefty price tag; you can make your own for a fraction of the cost.

2 cups (500 ml) borax (desert salt)
½ cup (125 ml) fine ground sea salt
½ cup (125 ml) baking soda (soda ash)
¼ cup (50 ml) white clay
½ cup (125 ml) dried herb of your choice
10 drops essential oil

Yield: Approximately 3¾ cups (925 ml)

To make:

1. In a large bowl, mix together the salts, baking soda, and clay.

2. Prepare the dried herb by powdering in a spice mill, crumbling by hand, or leaving whole if you prefer (see box below on preparing herbs).

3. Add the dried herbs to the salt mix, stirring with a wire whisk.

4. Scent the mixture using the essential oil of your choice. (Be sure to choose oils that are safe for external use.) Do not overscent; excess oil results in a clumpy, unattractive product — trust me.

5. Mix well with a wire whisk, then cover with a towel.

6. Leave overnight to fix the scent.

7. In the morning, thoroughly mix again and package.

To use:

Add ¼ to ½ cup (50 to 125 ml) sand to a tubful of warm water.

A NOTE ON PREPARING HERBS

Crush the dried herbs for bath sand as finely or coarsely as you like, or you can even leave them whole. Powdering is the best idea for anyone with temperamental plumbing; if you leave the herbs whole, it's probably a good idea to package the finished mixture in a small muslin bag for use in the tub. This will also make tub cleaning easier than if you throw the sand freely into the tub.

HEALING SALT CRYSTALS

If your health practitioner has recommended Epsom salts baths for your aching bones, this recipe is for you. It is very similar to the Fine Crystal Bathing Sand recipe, but has a coarser texture.

1 cup (250 ml) borax (desert salt)

2 cups (500 ml) Epsom salts

½ cup (125 ml) coarse sea salt

¼ cup (50 ml) baking soda

¼ cup (50 ml) white clay

½ cup (125 ml) dried herb of your choice

10 drops essential oil

Yield: 4 cups (1 liter)

To make:

1. In a large bowl, mix together the borax, salts, baking soda, and clay.

2. Prepare the dried herb by powdering in a spice mill, crumbling by hand, or leaving whole if you prefer (see box on preparing herbs).

3. Add the dried herbs to the salt mix, stirring with a wire whisk.

4. Scent the mix using the essential oil of your choice. (Be sure to choose oils that are safe for external use.) Do not overscent; excess oil will result in a clumpy, unattractive product.

5. Mix well with wire whisk, then cover with a towel.

6. Leave overnight to fix the scent.

7. In the morning, thoroughly mix again and package.

To use:

Add ¼ to ½ cup (50 to 125 ml) sand to a tubful of warm water.

PACKAGING BATH SALTS

Package salts in pretty jars, zipseal bags, muslin bags, or small seed-type envelopes. You can decorate any of these packages with stickers, ribbons or raffia, and bows, or have your children draw pictures on the envelopes before filling.

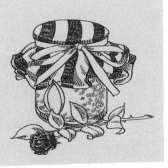

BUBBLE BATHS

Bubble baths are great fun for the kid in all of us. Unfortunately, they can leave your skin dry and itchy. Be sure to rinse thoroughly with clear water when finished bathing. If you are prone to dry, itchy skin, rinse in vinegar or lemon juice combined with water to counter the alkalinity of the soap and return your skin to its more natural pH, which is slightly acidic. The citrus and kiddie bubbles that follow are based on a recipe in Janice Cox's book, *Natural Beauty at Home*.

CITRUS BUBBLES

1 lemon
1 egg white
1 packet unflavored gelatin (¼ ounce [7 g])
1 tablespoon (15 ml) sesame, safflower, or canola oil
¼ cup (50 ml) unscented castile liquid soap
2 drops each lime, lemon, orange, and grapefruit essential oils

Yield: Makes enough bubbles for 1 bath

To make:
1. Juice the lemon and pour into a small container.
2. Lightly beat the egg white in a small bowl.
3. Fold the gelatin into the egg white.
4. In a bowl, combine all ingredients, including the lemon juice, and mix well.

To use:
1. Start running the water for your bath.
2. When the tub is half full of water, pour the Citrus Bubbles into the bath directly under the tap and mix well.
3. Slip into the tub as soon as the mix is poured to receive the full benefit of the aromas from the essential oils.
4. Rinse with cool water after bathing.

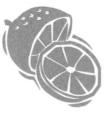

KIDDIE BUBBLES

This is a fun recipe for children and has none of the chemicals found in most commercial products.

1 egg white
2 packets unflavored gelatin (½ ounce [14 g])
⅓ cup (75 ml) liquid castile soap
1 tablespoon (15 ml) sesame oil
6 drops essential oil of orange or strawberry

Yield: Makes enough bubbles for 1 bath

To make:
1. Beat the egg white slightly.
2. Fold in the gelatin.
3. Pour all ingredients into a bowl and mix well.

To use:
1. Start running the water for your bath.
2. When the tub is half full of water, pour the Kiddie Bubbles into the bath directly under the tap and mix well.
3. Slip into the tub as soon as the mix is poured to receive the full benefit of the aromas from the essential oils.
4. Rinse with cool water after bathing.

SPICE ISLAND ESCAPE

Can't get away to the Spice Islands in the next week or so? Try this bath oil — it's the next best thing! This recipe is adapted from *The World Beauty Book* by Jessica Harris.

¼ cup (50 ml) sesame oil
⅛ cup (25 ml) cinnamon chips
5 whole cloves
1 large bay leaf, crumbled
Dash nutmeg or mace

Yield: 1 treatment

To make:
1. Place all ingredients in a glass jar. Let them steep for 1 week, shaking daily.
2. Strain the spices out of the oil using a fine mesh strainer.

To use:
1. Start filling the tub with water. When the tub is half full of water, pour the spicy sesame oil under the tap.
2. Slip into the tub as soon as the mix is poured to receive the full benefit of the scented oil.
3. Rinse with cool water after bathing.

VINEGAR HERBAL BATHS

In much the same way as you might make herbal vinegars for your salads, you can also create products that help restore the natural pH of your skin. Vinegar rinses are great diluted after bathing in alkaline soaps. Slightly acid baths are good for itchy skin. Vinegar rinses leave your hair shiny (see chapter 4).

ROSE PETAL VINEGAR BATH

Roses have been used for eons to enhance beauty and as symbols of love. I can't bear to pick my rose petals when the flowers are young; I always wait until the petals are almost ready to fall off naturally. Probably some of the medicinal and aromatic properties of the plant are lost, but they work fine for me and I get to enjoy the flowers longer. Any rose petals will work —wild roses or cultivated varieties — but please don't use your Valentine's Day bouquet, as commercial roses are heavily sprayed with pesticides.

2 cups (500 ml) fresh rose petals

1 quart (1 liter) apple cider vinegar

Yield: 2 baths

To make:
1. Collect fresh rose petals.
2. Spread the rose petals on paper towels and allow them to wilt overnight.
3. Pour vinegar into a saucepan.
4. Bring to a boil on medium heat.
5. Place the rose petals in a sterilized, wide-mouthed jar.
6. Pour the vinegar over the petals.
7. Cap the jar with a nonmetal lid and steep for 2 weeks.
8. Strain and bottle in sterilized vinegar bottles.
9. Cork or cap and decorate with stickers, raffia, and ribbons.

To use:
1. Begin drawing a tub of warm water.
2. When the tub is half full, add 2 cups (500 ml) of Rose Petal Vinegar.
3. Slip off your clothes and slip into the tub.
4. Relax for 10 to 20 minutes.
5. Rinsing with clear water is optional.

VENUS VINEGAR BATH

This recipe is dedicated to the goddess of love and the goddess present in every woman.

1 cup (250 ml) rose petals

1 cup (250 ml) lemon balm

1 cup (250 ml) calendula blossoms

1 cup (250 ml) comfrey leaves

2 quarts (2 liters) apple cider vinegar

Yield: 4 baths

To make:

1. Collect herbs and flowers fresh, if possible. If using dried, use half the suggested amounts.

2. Spread the herbs and flower petals on paper towels and allow them to wilt overnight.

3. The next day, pour vinegar into a saucepan.

4. Bring to a boil on medium heat.

5. Place the herbs and flower petals in a sterilized widemouthed jar.

6. Pour the vinegar over the petals.

7. Cap the jar with a nonmetal lid and steep for 2 weeks.

8. Strain and bottle in sterilized vinegar bottles.

9. Cork or cap and decorate with stickers, raffia, and ribbons.

To use:

1. Begin drawing a tub of warm water.

2. When the tub is half full, add 2 cups (500 ml) of Venus Vinegar.

3. Slip off your clothes and slip into the tub.

4. Relax for 10 to 20 minutes.

5. Rinsing with clear water is optional.

HERBAL INFUSION BATHS

An herbal infusion is basically a very strong herbal tea. The infusion is created by steeping herbs for 20 minutes up to 4 hours. (See page 4 for instructions on how to brew herbal tea.)

Any herbal tea blend you might drink will also work well in the bath. Don't limit yourself to these recipes; use them as a starting place for developing your own bath blends with your favorite herbs.

COMFREY INFUSION BATH

Comfrey is used externally for sprains, strains, and even broken bones. This recipe works best when made fresh, but it will keep 3 days in the refrigerator.

2 tablespoons (30 ml) fresh comfrey (1 tablespoon [15 ml] dried)
2 cups (500 ml) boiling water

Yield: 1 bath treatment

To make:
1. Place the comfrey in a 1-pint (475-ml) jar.
2. Pour boiling water over the comfrey and steep, covered, for 20 minutes to 4 hours.
3. Strain out the herbs, reserving the liquid for the bath.

To use:
1. Add the 2 cups (500 ml) of herbal infusion to a tub half full of warm water.
2. Slip off your clothes and slip into the tub.
3. Relax in the tub for 10 to 20 minutes.
4. Rinse with clear, tepid water.
5. Pat dry.

APHRODITE'S PLEASURE BATH

This recipe is best used freshly made, but it will last 3 days in the refrigerator.

2 tablespoons (30 ml) fresh rose petals (1 tablespoon [15 ml] dried)

2 tablespoons (30 ml) fresh comfrey (1 tablespoon [15 ml] dried)

2 tablespoons (30 ml) fresh elderflowers (1 tablespoon [15 ml] dried)

2 cups (500 ml) boiling water

Yield: 1 treatment

To make:

1. Place the herbs in a 1-pint (475-ml) jar.

2. Pour boiling water over the herbs and steep, covered, for 20 minutes to 4 hours.

3. Strain the liquid for use in the bath.

To use:

1. Add the 2 cups (500 ml) of herbal tea to a tub half full of warm water.

2. Slip off your clothes and slip into the tub.

3. Relax in the tub for 10 to 20 minutes.

4. Rinse with tepid water.

5. Pat dry.

MILK BATHS

Milk baths were a favorite of Cleopatra. The fat of the milk is nourishing to the skin, especially to dry skin. Those with oily skin may choose lower-fat varieties or even nonfat milk powder.

EASY MILK BATH

1. Add 1 quart (1 liter) of milk to a tub half full of warm water.

2. Slip in and relax for 10 to 20 minutes.

3. Rinse with cool water.

4. Pat dry.

COMPRESSES AND POULTICES

Compresses and poultices are techniques for bathing small areas where you may have a breakout, cut, bruise, sprain, or other injury. Using compresses or fomentation is a great way to speed the healing process.

COMFREY COMPRESS FOR SPRAINS AND STRAINS

2 tablespoons (30 ml) fresh herbs (1 tablespoon [15 ml] dried)
2 cups (500 ml) boiling water
Clean cloth, either linen, cotton, or gauze

Yield: 1 treatment

To make:
1. Place the herbs in a clean, 20-ounce (567-g) jar.
2. Pour boiling water over the herbs and steep, covered, for 5 to 20 minutes.
3. Strain the herbs from the infusion and pour remaining liquid into a saucepan.
To use:
1. Reheat the infusion on a low simmer.
2. Remove from heat and put the cloth in the liquid.
3. While still hot, remove the cloth and wring it so it does not drip too much.
4. Place the cloth, as hot as possible, over the affected area. Heat enhances the action of the herbs, so using a hot water bottle to keep the compress warm for 20 minutes is helpful. Be sure to throw the cloth away when you are finished with it.

MAKING A POULTICE FROM A SOCK

Poultices are often used to soothe ankles, wrists, elbows, and feet. An easy way to get all of the healing benefits of the herbs and heat without a lot of fuss and muss is to make a poultice using a cotton sock.

1. Cut the sock above the foot portion.

2. Place 1 cup (250 ml) of dried herbs in a small bowl.

3. Pour ½ cup (125 ml) of boiling water over the herbs.

4. Using a strainer, scoop up the hot herbal material, allow the water to drain, and pour the herbs into the toe area of the sock. The herbs will fill approximately one-third of the sock.

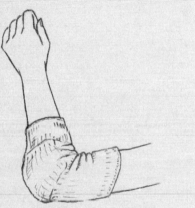

5. Wrap the rest of the sock around the toe portion — poultice — and place it on the sore or sprained elbow, ankle, wrist, or foot.

6. Use the elasticized portion of the sock to secure the poultice in place. Leave the poultice on until it cools.

EASY POULTICE

A poultice is similar to a compress but instead of the liquid infusion, the solid plant material is used. Plantain, comfrey, lavender, even cabbage leaves work well. Often the plants growing wild in your yard are useful.

1 cup (250 ml) fresh or ½ cup (125 ml) dried herbs of your choice

¼ cup (50 ml) hot water or hot apple cider

Yield: 1 treatment

To make:
1. If you are using fresh plant material, bruise the leaves or tear into small pieces.
2. Add just enough hot water or hot apple cider vinegar to dampen the herbs.

To use:
Place the herbs directly on the skin or in layers of gauze, which will then be applied to the affected area.

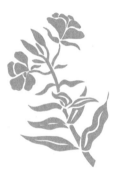

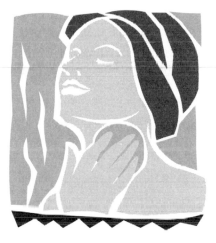

Herbs for the Feet and Hands

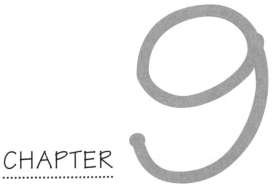

CHAPTER 9

If you stop for a moment to think about how much your feet and hands do for you each day, you'll appreciate the value of time spent nurturing and caring for these hard-working extremities. I've included recipes to nourish and care for the nails, making them stronger and less brittle, as well as recipes for softening and moisturizing the skin of the feet and hands.

Gardeners often have abused hands. If you're an herb lover, as I am, you probably get your hands in dirt as often as you can. People ask if I have a green thumb — actually, I have a brown thumbnail and fingernails! Anyone who works with their hands, from plasterers to masons to artists, will benefit from the formulas in this chapter. They're designed to help counter the drying effects of all the things our hands manage to find their way into.

EQUIPMENT FOR HAND AND NAIL CARE

You are probably familiar with many of the tools of the trade for hand and foot care. All of these items can be purchased at a pharmacy or health and beauty store. I have had a little

A DIET FOR HEALTHY NAILS

Eating a healthy diet is especially important for healthy nails. Too little protein can make your nails brittle and dull. Deficiencies in vitamins and minerals can also show up in the nails. Be sure to eat those leafy green vegetables and fresh fruits.

Herbal tea can also improve your fingernails over time. Drinking 1 to 3 cups (250 to 750 ml) per day, you should notice improvement in 3 weeks. Yes, iced tea works just as well as hot.

The best herbal teas for healthy nails include borage, chamomile, nettle, oat straw, peppermint, and rose hips.

more trouble finding a nail buffer, but it's worth the search, since it helps natural nails glow. Following is a list of the tools you need.

For nail treatments:
- Emery board (not a metal file)
- Nail clippers
- Orange stick
- Finger bowls
- Hand basin (large enough to submerge both hands simultaneously)
- Hand towel
- White fingernail pencil
- Nail buffer

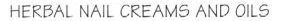

For foot treatments:
- Toenail clippers
- Pumice stone
- Basin

HERBAL NAIL CREAMS AND OILS

Quite a while ago, I met a woman at my workplace who had the most fabulous fingernails. I assumed they must be fake, but found out otherwise when I asked her about them. She told me her secret to long, healthy nails — a small container of an oil mixture that she had purchased commercially and used faithfully every day. Immediately, I went out and purchased the fingernail-polish-size bottle of oil, which cost close to ten dollars. It's quite an ingenious little product; works well, and is all natural. It even helps to dry nail polish.

I didn't think about the price too much at the time, since beauty products can be expensive. But when I got the product home and read the ingredients, I thought, why would ½ ounce (14 g) of this mixture cost nearly ten dollars when I can buy an

8-ounce (227-g) bottle of each ingredient for less than five dollars apiece? The answer is, of course, that the merchant is charging for the cost involved in mixing them together, packaging them in a pretty bottle, advertising, and selling retail. You can avoid paying those high costs by making your own, quite simply. Who knows, maybe you will develop an even better recipe than this one and make your fortune with it!

FABULOUS FINGERNAILS OIL

Nail dryness and brittleness are often the cause of nail breakage — this recipe can help!

1 teaspoon (5 ml) almond oil
1 teaspoon (5 ml) apricot kernel oil
1 teaspoon (5 ml) castor oil
1 teaspoon (5 ml) grapeseed oil
1 teaspoon (5 ml) olive oil
3 drops vitamin E oil
2 drops frankincense essential oil
2 drops benzoin resin

Yield: 2-month supply

To make:
1. Combine all oils and resin in a small amber glass bottle (Boston round) and mix thoroughly by shaking.
2. Keep refrigerated between uses.

To condition nails:
1. Using a cotton swab, apply liberally to the fingernail and cuticle.
2. Massage gently into the fingernail and cuticle.

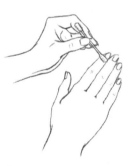

To use as a nail polish dryer:
1. Recycle a nail polish brush by cleaning it with nail polish remover and then soap and water. (You may be able to purchase a single new brush at a health and beauty store.)
2. Apply a thin coat of oil gently over just-applied nail polish, using smooth, even strokes.
3. Allow to air-dry.

HORSETAIL NAIL CREAM

This cream is especially good for nourishing and protecting the nails. Horsetail, considered a weed, is high in silica, which is found in healthy hair and nails. Make this recipe in the spring, when horsetail is in bloom. Get out your plant identification books and go out and gather it yourself. I think horsetail looks like a miniature (4-inch [10-cm]) Christmas tree. In a pinch, you can use dried horsetail. Benzoin gum resin is great for the nail bed and cuticles, conditioning where you need it most. These make great gifts.

1 cup (250 ml) fresh
   or ½ cup (125 ml)
   dried horsetail
1¼ cups (300 ml)
   olive oil
2 tablespoons
   (30 ml) beeswax
10 drops vitamin E oil
5 drops benzoin resin
30 ¼-ounce (7-gram)
   containers with lids

Yield: Thirty ¼-ounce
(7-gram) containers

To make:
1. Place the fresh horsetail on a towel and allow it to wilt overnight.
2. In a double boiler, steep the horsetail in olive oil over low heat for 3 hours.
3. Grate the beeswax.
4. Strain the plant material out of the oil completely, then pour the oil back into the double boiler. Add the grated beeswax.
5. Heat the mixture until the beeswax melts completely, then remove from heat.
6. Quickly add the vitamin E oil and benzoin gum resin.
7. Pour into dainty ¼-ounce (7-gram) containers or jars and decorate, if desired.
To use:
1. Place your thumb into the container, coating it liberally with nail cream.
2. Systematically massage the cream into each fingernail and cuticle bed.
3. Use twice daily and watch your fingernails improve.

PAPAYA CUTICLE SOAK

This recipe is great for hangnail sufferers. Papaya contains an enzyme that softens and dissolves the undesired cuticle. Regular care of the nails can help to eliminate cuticle problems, even for those who work their hands hard.

2 tablespoons (30 ml) papaya juice
2 tablespoons (30 ml) wheat germ oil
1 teaspoon (5 ml) olive oil

Yield: 1 treatment

To make:
1. In a blender, combine the juice and wheat germ oil. Run blender on the highest setting for 2 minutes.
To use:
1. Pour juice mixture into a small finger bowl.
2. Measure olive oil into a separate small dish.
3. Soak each hand in the juice mixture for 5 minutes, then rinse with tepid water.
4. Dip an orange stick into the olive oil, then use it to push back the cuticle on each finger.
5. Massage the olive oil into the cuticle.

GELATIN NAIL SOAK

Gelatin is another ingredient that helps build healthy nails and hair. Eating gelatin or taking gelatin supplements improves fingernail strength. External use of gelatin is also helpful.

½ packet gelatin
½ cup (125 ml) boiling water

Yield: 1 treatment

To make:
1. Place gelatin in a small glass bowl and pour boiling water over it. Mix well.
2. Allow gelatin mixture to cool to just warm.
To use:
1. While the mixture is still warm, soak your fingertips in it for 5 minutes.
2. Remove fingertips from bowl and massage the gelatin that remains on your fingers into the nail and nail bed.
3. Rinse with warm water.

HERBAL NAIL COLOR

Do you like the look of nail color but abhor the odor of commercial nail polish? Try henna or alkanet nail color, and buff for a subtle but fashionable look without the aroma.

ALKANET ROOT NAIL OIL

Alkanet root is known for its ability to color oils. It is a great addition to lip gloss and nail color because it has emollient properties as well. Alkanet can be grown in your garden, where you can enjoy the pretty violet flowers before using the root. Ask for seeds at your garden shop. Vary the amount of alkanet — use a little to achieve a blush pink color; use more for darker shades.

½ teaspoon (2 ml) alkanet root

3 tablespoons (45 ml) olive oil

¼ teaspoon (1 ml) beeswax

2 drops vitamin E oil

Yield: Several treatments; good for 1 year if refrigerated

To make:
1. Combine the olive oil and alkanet root in a double boiler.
2. Strain out the alkanet root with a fine mesh strainer, pouring the oil back into the double boiler.
3. Add the beeswax and heat until it melts.
4. Add the vitamin E to the oil, mix, and pour into a small dish or container.

To use:
1. Dip a small brush into the oil and paint your nails, being careful to avoid getting any of the mixture on the surrounding skin.
2. Allow the oil to dry, then reapply.
3. You may want to reapply several times to get a deeper red color.
4. Refrigerate unused portion.

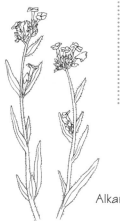

Alkanet

HENNA NAIL PASTE

Henna is not just for the hair — it can also be used to color nails naturally. Experiment with all the different shades to find one that complements your coloring. I love the tawny, earthy tone of brown henna. Orange henna and the black hennas also create interesting shades. Arab women use henna for spiritual protection and to bring prosperity.

1 tablespoon (15 ml) henna
1 tablespoon (15 ml) water
2 drops vitamin E oil

Yield: 1 treatment

To make:
1. Place the henna in a small dish and pour water over it.
2. Add the vitamin E and mix to form a paste.

To use:
1. While the paste is still warm, use a small brush to carefully apply paste to the fingernails only. Wash off any spills on your hands as soon as they occur or you will end up with colorful skin.
2. Allow henna to dry on the nails for at least 20 minutes, or until completely dry.
3. Rinse hands with warm water.
4. Buff nails with nail buffer.

MEHNDI OR HENNA TATTOOS

If you have some leftover henna, try your hand at creating temporary tattoos for kids (or yourself, if that's your thing!). Egyptian and Indian women use henna to paint intricate designs on their hands, a long-standing cultural tradition. Use a toothpick to create fine line drawings. Be sure to let one color of henna dry before applying another color or they will bleed together. *Note:* The henna will take a few weeks to totally wash off.

HAND-SOFTENING CREAMS

These recipes are especially nice for chapped hands caused by overexposure or by working with drying ingredients. In the winter be sure to wear gloves and drink enough water each day.

HAPPY HANDS HAND CREAM

Everyone loves this cream, but it is especially good for dry skin. Note: The proportions in this recipe are designed for success when combined in a standard kitchen blender; a food processor will not work.

Because of spoilage problems due to rancidity, unused jars of cream must be refrigerated. Package the cream in containers that are opaque or dark to protect them from the destabilizing effects of light. I keep one cream out on my vanity and the rest take up space in my refrigerator.

⅓ cup (75 ml) grapeseed oil

⅓ cup (75 ml) olive oil

⅓ cup (75 ml) coconut oil

1 tablespoon (15 ml) zinc oxide paste

1 teaspoon (5 ml) cocoa butter

1 tablespoon (15 ml) beeswax

⅓ cup (75 ml) orange blossom water

⅓ cup (75 ml) distilled water

⅓ cup (75 ml) aloe vera gel

20 drops vitamin E oil

5 drops essential oil of orange blossom

5 drops essential oil of frankincense

Yield: 15 1-ounce (25-gram) opaque jars

To make:

1. In a double boiler, melt the grapeseed, olive, and coconut oils; zinc oxide paste; cocoa butter; and beeswax.

2. Once the beeswax is melted, pour the oil mixture into a glass measuring cup, preferably one with a spout.

3. Let cool to room temperature for approximately 1 hour.

4. Set up your 15 clean 1-ounce (25-gram) jars on the edge of your counter for easy pouring.

5. Combine the orange blossom and distilled waters, aloe vera gel, and vitamin E and the essential oils in the blender and turn to the highest speed for a minute or two.

6. While the blender is still going, slowly drizzle the cooled oils into the vortex of the waters.

7. Listen to the blender; when it chokes, the water and oil have combined. Turn off the blender.

8. Pour cream into jars and decorate with stickers, ribbon, or labels.

HONEY PASTE

This formula is excellent for softening the most abused hands. It contains ingredients that are emollient and exfoliating at the same time, thus working to remove dry skin while softening the new skin. This recipe can also be used on the feet. It is best applied at bedtime, covered with gloves made of natural fiber, and then left on to work all night.

1 tablespoon (15 ml) almonds
1 tablespoon (15 ml) oatmeal
1 tablespoon (15 ml) zinc oxide paste
1 egg yolk
1 tablespoon (15 ml) honey
1 pair soft kid or cotton gloves

Yield: 1 treatment

To make:
1. In a coffee grinder or spice mill, roughly grind the almonds and the oatmeal, leaving some grit.
2. In a bowl, combine the ground almonds and oatmeal with the zinc oxide paste, egg yolk, and honey, stirring well.

To use:
1. Rub the paste into your hands.
2. Recruit someone to help you put on gloves over your paste-covered hands.
3. Go to sleep for the night, allowing the paste to work its magic. *Note:* You may not want to sleep on your best sheets and bedding if you are concerned about dripping or staining.
4. In the morning, remove the gloves, rinse your hands with cool water, and feel the softness.

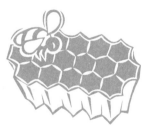

HERBAL PARAFFIN HAND TREATMENTS

This recipe is similar to those you might be treated with in a spa salon. Prepare it in a large, 3-pound (1-kilogram) coffee can so you can dip your entire hand into it, and your elbows, too. If you don't want to make that much, prepare a smaller amount and apply to the hands with a paintbrush. Wax treatments help the skin to absorb moisture, and are especially helpful for dry hands. Frankincense has cell-regenerating properties.

24 ounces (678 g) paraffin wax

4 ounces (113 g) beeswax

1 cup (250 ml) apricot kernel oil

20 drops vitamin E oil

8 drops frankincense essential oil

8 drops lavender essential oil

Yield: 12 hand treatments

To make:

1. In a double boiler, melt the waxes and apricot kernel oil on low heat.

2. Once melted, remove from heat and pour the wax mixture into a clean, large (3-pound [1-kilogram]) coffee can. Be sure the can does not have any sharp edges.

3. Add the vitamin E and essential oils and stir well with a chopstick or spoon.

To use:

1. First apply the Happy Hands Hand Cream (see recipe on page 155) or another hand cream thoroughly and liberally, massaging the cream into your hands.

2. While the wax is still warm but not too hot, dip one hand and then the other into the wax.

3. Allow the wax to air-cool and harden, approximately 20 minutes.

4. Gently peel off the paraffin and discard. Note: You can store the leftover wax right in the coffee can by placing the lid on it, but be sure to use it within 1 year. To use again, reheat and melt in a water bath. You may choose to add more essential oil and vitamin E, as they will dissipate with reheating.

HERBAL FOOTBATHS AND SOAKS

Many herbs are delightful to use in a footbath, and footbaths are delightful because you enjoy an aromatherapy session at the same time. Any herbs that you might use for external use or drink as tea are generally good for baths. The herbs are prepared the same way as herbal infusions (see page 142). Footbaths are simple to prepare, and your feet definitely deserve some pampering.

> **CAUTION**
>
> The treatments presented in this chapter are beneficial for addressing a wide range of health concerns. However, you should consult your doctor before engaging in the treatments, especially if you have varicose veins or circulation or heart problems.

HERBAL FOOTBATH

2 cups (500 ml) fresh herbs of your choice (1 cup [250 ml] dried)
Boiling water

Yield: 1 treatment

To make:

1. Select desired herb or herb combination (see box) and place in a 1-quart (1-liter) jar.
2. Pour boiling water over the herbs, cover tightly, and allow to steep for 20 minutes.

To use:

1. Strain the liquid from the herbs (called an herbal infusion) into a foot basin.
2. Add warm water to achieve the level and temperature desired. Use care in your choice of temperature: 100° to 110°F is best.
3. Submerge your feet and relax for 10 minutes.
4. Enlist a friend to rub your feet while they are in the water and to pat them dry when finished, or you can do this for yourself.

OLIVE OIL SOFTENING SOAK

Also great for the fingernails, this recipe contains olive oil infused with sage, horsetail, and red clover. It is helpful for brittle nails and for calluses. I like to make enough for the feet and use the rest on my hands and fingertips, but you can make a smaller batch just for your hands. For sanitary purposes, make a fresh batch for each individual.

3 ounces (85 g) fresh sage

3 ounces (85 g) fresh red clover

2 cups (500 ml) olive oil

3 ounces (85 g) fresh horsetail

5 drops vitamin E oil

5 drops vanilla essential oil

1 16-ounce (454-gram) amber-colored bottle (Boston round) or two 8-ounce (227-gram) bottles

Yield: 2 cups (500 ml)

To make:

1. Gather the fresh herbs and lay them on a paper towel to wilt overnight. (This allows for any dew or water on the plant material to evaporate, thereby protecting your oil from contamination.)

2. The next day, combine the oil and wilted herbs in a double boiler.

3. Simmer on low for 4 hours.

4. Strain the plant material, reserving the oil.

5. Add the vitamin E oil and essential oil to this mixture.

6. Pour into the amber bottle(s).

To use:

1. Pour 1 cup of oil into a warm-water footbath.

2. Submerse both feet and relax for 10 minutes.

3. Enlist a friend to rub your feet while they are in the water and to pat them dry when finished, or you can do this part yourself.

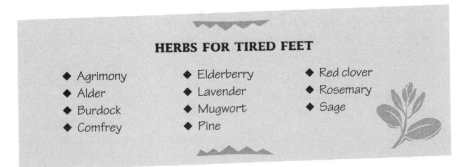

HERBS FOR TIRED FEET

- Agrimony
- Alder
- Burdock
- Comfrey
- Elderberry
- Lavender
- Mugwort
- Pine
- Red clover
- Rosemary
- Sage

HOT AND COLD FOOTBATH

Hot and cold stimulation is great for the entire body and especially help-ful to the feet. Jethro Kloss recommends the treatment for a myriad of health problems (see *Back to Eden*). I like using it after ice skating. You will be amazed at how good this simple procedure feels. If you suffer from cir-culation or other health problems, be sure to check with your doctor before doing this treatment.

In place of the hot water in this recipe, you can use the herbal infu-sion or olive oil soak (see pages 158–159) for the hot bath and thus receive the benefit of the herbs and oils.

2 foot basins
Hot water to fill basin
2/3 full
Cold water to fill basin
2/3 full

Yield: 1 treatment

To make:
1. Heat hot-water bath to 100° to 110°F.
2. Make cold-water bath 50°F.
To use:
1. Starting with the basin of hot water, submerse your feet for 5 minutes.
2. Remove your feet from the hot water and place them in the cold-water basin for 2 minutes.
3. Go back to the hot and repeat as desired, being sure to finish with the cold.
4. Pat dry.

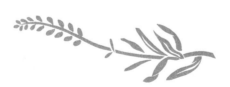

HERBAL FOOT SCRUBS

Any number of ingredients can be used for making foot scrubs. The recipes for facial scrubs in chapter 5 are almost as effective for the feet as they are for the face. You may have heard of the benefits of walking in sand with bare feet: Sand can also be used as an ingredient in foot scrubs. Avocado pit meal and avocado skins are great, too, and you get to make use of parts you would just be throwing out otherwise.

While you might use facial recipes on your feet, I don't recommend using foot scrub recipes on the delicate skin on your face and body. They're best for the tougher skin of the feet, elbows, and knees.

A WALK ON THE BEACH

1 cup (250 ml) sand (coarseness of your choice)
1 tablespoon (15 ml) sea salt
1 tablespoon (15 ml) powdered dulse
1 tablespoon (15 ml) powdered kelp
1 cup (250 ml) olive oil
2 foot basins

Yield: 2 treatments

To make:
1. Place the sand, salt, and seaweeds in a bowl.
2. Pour the olive oil over the mixture, mixing well.

To use:
1. Place your feet in a foot basin. Massage the sand mixture into both feet, giving special care to your heels.
2. Move feet to second basin and rinse your feet with cool water.
3. Repeat the treatment, and rinse again in cool water.
4. Pat dry.

AVOCADO SKIN SOFTENER

Avocados help soften and remove calluses. Each part of the avocado has a different use. The ground pit makes a wonderful emollient scrub, the pulp is a rich moisturizer that is especially good for dry skin, and the skin of the fruit contains a potent cosmetic oil. Application of this formula will dissolve dead skin and make your feet feel satiny smooth.

1 avocado pit
½ avocado
¼ cup (50 ml) cornmeal
1 tablespoon (15 ml) sea salt

Yield: 1 treatment

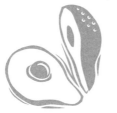

To make:

1. Dry out the avocado pit for a few days, then break into several pieces.

2. In a spice mill or coffee grinder, grind the pit to make gritty avocado pit meal.

3. Reserving its skin, mash the ½ avocado with the cornmeal, ¼ cup (50 ml) avocado pit meal, and sea salt.

To use:

1. In a foot basin, gently massage the mixture into your feet in a circular motion, starting with the toes.

2. Massage the scrub into the ball of each foot working into and around all the little bones there.

3. Massage and stroke the arches.

4. With a bit more pressure, work on the heels and the outside of the foot.

5. Massage the ankles and the tops of the feet.

6. Rinse with tepid water.

7. With the inner (sticky) side of the avocado skin, rub the heel and any other callused areas including your knees, elbows, and hands. Do not rinse off. Massage the oil into the skin with your hands in gentle, circular motions.

8. At first your skin may seem green, but keep massaging. Soon you'll feel the abrasive effects, then the moisturizing effects.

PUMICE FOOT EXFOLIATION

You can purchase pumice stones at any pharmacy. I like to use mine while bathing, but a pumice stone scrub can also be combined with any of the preceding foot treatments. A pumice stone treatment accompanied by a reflexology rub makes a much appreciated "hands-on" gift for a friend or loved one.

Pumice stone
Soap
Water

To use:

1. Soften your feet by soaking them in water or an herb bath for a few minutes.

2. Wash the feet thoroughly.

3. In a circular motion, rub the pumice stone around all parts of the feet.

4. Rinse with tepid water.

5. Pat dry.

REFLEXOLOGY FOOT MASSAGE

Reflexology is a method for activating the healing powers of the body through massage techniques applied to the feet (or hands). More than just a simple foot rub (not to diminish the value of that) however, reflexology is a systematic approach to the feet, taking into account any health problems. It is based on the principle that there are energy zones (referred to as meridians by the acupuncturist or Chinese healer) that run through the body and the feet. These areas reflect or "reflex" and correspond to all the organs, glands, and other parts of the whole body. Similar to the concept of a hologram, which always contains the whole, by working on the corresponding spots on the feet or the hands, you can affect the whole body.

For a more in-depth appreciation of reflexology, consult your bookstore or library. There are also training programs specifically set up to teach and certify individuals in the art and science of reflexology. Many manicurists and pedicurists are familiar with the techniques; you may want to indulge in a professional treatment with one of them and consult about how to practice at home.

DEODORIZING AND CURATIVE FOOT TREATMENTS

Our feet do much for us each day and, sadly, they are often the most neglected part of our bodies. Be sure to pamper your feet, and treat them to footbaths, foot rubs, and invigorating foot powders every now and then.

HERBAL FOOT POWDER

This powder is easy to make, at a fraction of the cost of commercial products, and contains only all-natural ingredients — how can you lose? The elderberry helps reduce fatigue. Some of the old herbals recommend putting elder flowers or leaves in your shoes. Lovage is one of my favorite aromatics and is a natural deodorant. Note: This powder may also be used as a body powder (see recipe on page 173).

½ cup (125 ml) dried elder flowers or leaves
½ cup (125 ml) dried lovage
1 cup (250 ml) white clay
2 cups (500 ml) cornstarch
8 drops peppermint essential oil
Powder cylinders or a recycled powder puff and container

Yield: 4 cups (1 liter)

To make:

1. In a spice mill or coffee grinder, grind the elder flowers and then the lovage to a fine powder.

2. In a large bowl, combine all dry ingredients, mixing with a wire whisk.

3. Scent with essential oil, and again mix with the wire whisk.

4. Allow mixture to sit overnight, covered with a towel, to fix the scent.

5. In the morning, mix again with a wire whisk.

6. Package in powder cylinders.

To use:

1. Sprinkle powder in your shoes before putting them on in the morning.

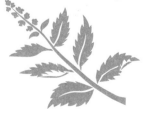

CORN CURE

1 garlic clove for each
corn

Yield: 1 treatment

To make:
1. Roast garlic cloves.
To use:
1. While hot, apply a whole garlic clove directly to a corn.
2. Place a bandage over each corn and garlic clove.
3. Repeat application for 3 to 4 days, until corns loosen and fall off. (You'll keep vampires away at the same time!)

ATHLETE'S FOOT CURE

You won't find this cure in any luxury spas, but it won't cost you a dime and is highly effective. Urine, or urea, is slightly acidic and is an ingredient in many beauty products, valued for its healing properties and the fact that it is closer to the natural pH of the skin. Uncontaminated urine is highly sanitary, pure, and antiseptic. It was used on battlefields for surgery and works particularly well on jellyfish stings. Some ancient cultures bathed in urine as a beauty ritual. Eastern cultures use urine for beauty and for healing. Also works well on warts, including plantar's warts.

1 cup (250 ml) urine
from the person
being treated
1 gallon (4 liters)
warm water

Yield: 1 treatment

To make:
1. In a foot basin, combine the urine and warm water.
To use:
1. Soak feet for 20 minutes.
2. Rinse with cool water.
Variation: If you cannot bring yourself to use urine, substitute ½ cup lemon juice or apple cider vinegar. This combination will require more frequent treatments, but it is effective because of the acidity. Nonalkaline soap is also helpful, as is a black walnut hull herbal infusion footbath (see recipe on page 158 and substitute black walnut hulls, which have antifungal properties, for the herbs).

HERBAL FOOT CIRCULATION POWDER

A friend got a pretty bad case of frostbite and almost had to quit his job, working outdoors in Colorado in winter. Using this powder increased the circulation to his feet. Not only was he able to keep his job, but also his feet, which he had been told would always be whitish and part dead, regained their natural pink color.

If you have circulation problems due to diabetes or other problems, ask your doctor about the use of this recipe. Similar to the heating products used for increasing circulation and reducing arthritis pain, the cayenne powder is slightly irritating. This is a great product to keep in your survival kit if you live in an area with cold winters. In a winter wisdom class that I teach, I suggest people keep a small amount of cayenne, along with a blanket, in their car just in case they break down and are stranded on a wintry night. The cayenne can be used to sprinkle in your shoes and in extremities that might be prone to frostbite (e.g., fingers, nose, ears).

1 cup (250 ml) white clay
2 cups (500 ml) cornstarch
3 tablespoons (45 ml) cayenne pepper

Yield: 3 cups (750 ml)

To make:
1. Combine all ingredients in a large bowl, mixing with a wire whisk.
2. Package in powder cylinders.

To use:
1. Sprinkle in your shoes.
2. Wear socks to protect from possible skin irritation.
3. Wash hands thoroughy after applying, as it can be painful if you get it in your eyes. If you should get some in your eyes, flush your eyes thoroughly with water.

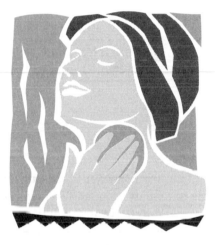

Herbal Hygiene

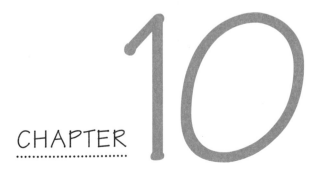

CHAPTER 10

Throughout the centuries, people in various cultures have used herbal products to stay fresh and clean. Herbal teas have traditionally been used for internal cleansing. Herbal mouthwashes and gargles keep breath fresh and can also help with oral hygiene. Herbal tooth powders are easy to make and leave the teeth feeling smooth. A variety of aromatic herbs lend themselves to scenting body powders. Herbal underarm deodorant can help to keep you feeling fresh.

HERBAL TEAS

Herbal beverages can help keep the body fresh and clean. Drinking eight glasses of water daily also helps keep the body fresh by helping it excrete toxins.

BODY-FRESHENING TEA

Almost any herbal tea or infusion will help freshen your body, but the ones listed here are notable for their body odor–defying qualities. Increase the amount of herbs and water proportionally to brew as many cups as you desire. It is best to make it fresh daily, but it can be refrigerated for two days.

This recipe can easily be doubled or tripled. Simply use the basic ratio of 1 tablespoon fresh or 1 teaspoon dried herbs for each 8 ounces of water and tea desired.

8 ounces (227 g) water

1 tablespoon (15 ml) of one of the following fresh herbs (1 teaspoon [5 ml] dried):
  Lovage
  Sagebrush
  Peppermint
  Cleavers
  Thyme

Yield: 1 cup

To make:
1. Bring the water to a boil.
2. Place the herbs in a jar and pour the boiling water over them; cover.
3. Steep flowers briefly for 5 minutes; steep leafy material for 20 minutes. Strain out herbs and reserve liquid.

To use:
1. Drink 3 cups per day for best results.

HERBAL MOUTHWASH AND GARGLE

Herbal mouthwash and gargle is yet another product that is easy to make and use, and it doesn't have any of the chemicals common in many commercial products. Do remember that serious breath problems are often the result of poor digestion. Consult with your physician if in doubt.

CINNAMON SPICE MOUTHWASH

1 tablespoon (15 ml) cinnamon chips
1 tablespoon (15 ml) whole cloves
1 teaspoon (5 ml) anise seed
1 teaspoon (5 ml) ground nutmeg
1 cup (250 ml) vodka

Yield: 16 treatments

To make:
1. Place all the spices in a clean glass jar.
2. Pour the vodka over the spices, cap, and shake daily for the next 2 weeks.
3. Strain and pour into a dark amber bottle.
To use:
1. This mouthwash is concentrated. Use 1 tablespoon mouthwash dissolved in 1 cup (250 ml) water.
2. Gargle as usual.
3. Rinse with clear, cool water.

DIET FOR A FRESH-SMELLING BODY

Diet is a major contributor to body odor, as are hormonal fluctuations. A vegetarian diet or one high in fruits and vegetables reduces body odor because chlorophyll, a substance naturally found in green plants, helps control the bacteria that cause body odor. Parsley, beet greens, and lovage have a cleansing effect on both the breath and body odors.

MINTY MOUTHWASH

½ cup (125 ml)
  spearmint
½ cup (125 ml)
  peppermint
1 cup (250 ml) white
  wine

Yield: 16 treatments

To make:
1. Place the herbs in a clean glass jar.
2. Pour the white wine over the herbs, cap, and shake daily for the next 2 weeks.
3. Strain and pour into a dark amber bottle.

To use:
1. This mouthwash is concentrated. Use 1 tablespoon mouthwash dissolved in 1 cup (250 ml) water.
2. Gargle as usual.
3. Rinse with clear, cool water.

LAVENDER-PEPPERMINT MOUTH RINSE

Searching for a nonalcoholic product? Look no further. Since there is no alcohol to preserve this recipe, it must be made fresh each time.

1 tablespoon (15 ml)
  fresh lavender (1 tea-
  spoon [5 ml] dried)
1 tablespoon (15ml)
  peppermint (1 tea-
  spoon [5 ml] dried)
1 cup (250 ml) water

Yield: 1 treatment

To make:
1. Bring the water to a boil.
2. Add the herbs to a clean glass jar.
3. Pour the boiling water over the herbs and let steep for 30 minutes.
4. Strain.

To use:
1. Gargle with the strong herbal tea.

BREATH-FRESHENING HERBS

Cloves, fennel seed, parsley, peppermint, spearmint, watercress, and wintergreen are useful to freshen the breath.

I like to chew on fresh wintergreen, parsley, or the mints. The spices, fennel, and cloves can be used dried; simply chew on them. Use these herbs and spices in place of breath mints and avoid the added sugar and artificial sweeteners.

Factors that may contribute to chronic breath odor are inadequate diet and stomach and other health problems. Bad breath should be checked by a healthcare provider if it persists.

HERBAL TOOTH CARE

Tooth powders are fun and easy to make. The baking soda produces a naturally fresh, clean feeling in the mouth, while affecting its pH and making it less acidic.

HERBAL TOOTH POWDER

Myrrh powder is added to this recipe to help prevent periodontal disease. Baking soda, an ingredient in many commercial products, lessens the mouth's acidity. Raspberry leaf is good for the gums and mildly astringent. Tea tree oil is effective against gingivitis and plaque buildup; the yellow dock is cleansing.

½ cup (125 ml) baking soda

½ cup (125 ml) clay powder

1 teaspoon (5 ml) myrrh powder

1 teaspoon (5 ml) dried raspberry leaf

1 teaspoon (5 ml) dried yellow dock root

1 teaspoon (5 ml) flavoring herbs of your choice (fennel, peppermint, spearmint, wintergreen)

5 drops essential oil of tea tree

Yield: about 1 cup (250 ml)

To make:
1. Pour the baking soda and white clay powder into a medium-size mixing bowl.
2. In a spice mill or coffee grinder, grind the dried herbs into a powder.
3. Add all the dry ingredients, including the myrrh powder, to the baking soda–clay mixture.
4. Mix well with a wire whisk.
5. Add the tea tree oil, again mixing well.
6. Place a clean hand towel over the bowl, covering it completely.
7. Let sit overnight.
8. The next morning, mix well again with the wire whisk.
9. Package in an opaque widemouthed jar. It will last indefinitely if you keep moisture out of the package.
To use:
1. Wet your toothbrush, then sprinkle a small quantity of powder onto your brush.
2. Brush thoroughly and gently in an up-and-down motion.
3. Brush the tongue, too.
4. Rinse, and feel the freshness of your mouth.

STRAWBERRY TEETH WHITENER

This recipe leaves the teeth clean and shiny. Strawberries have been used through the centuries for tooth whitening.

3–6 ripe strawberries
1 teaspoon (5 ml) baking soda plus 1 teaspoon (5 ml)
1 teaspoon (5 ml) cream of tartar
1 cup water

Yield: 1 treatment

To make:
1. In a blender, puree the berries.
2. Pour the fruit into a small custard-size dish.

To use:
1. With your toothbrush or a cosmetic brush, paint a paste of the berries onto your teeth. Let sit on teeth for 5 minutes.
2. Add the baking soda and cream of tartar to the cup of water.
3. Swish the soda water around in your mouth.
4. Brush your teeth with plain baking soda.
5. Rinse with cool, clear water.

HERBAL BODY POWDER AND DEODORANTS

I don't recommend using antiperspirant; perspiration is a natural, and necessary, process in a healthy body. Natural deodorants like the following do not block the skin or clog the pores; they do alter the scent of perspiration and affect the bacteria that cause body odor.

HERBAL BODY POWDER

This powder is easy to make and at a fraction of the cost of commercial products. With only natural ingredients, how can you go wrong? Use it in place of deodorant or antiperspirant. It is also effective at preventing the chafing between the thighs that you may experience when bicycle riding or in hot, humid weather.

1 cup (250 ml) white clay

2 cups (500 ml) cornstarch

¼ cup (50 ml) powdered herb of your choice. (Lavender and rose are nice, but any aromatic will work.)

8 drops essential oil

Yield: Approximately 3 cups

To make:

1. Combine all dry ingredients in a large bowl, mixing with a wire whisk.

2. Scent with essential oil and cover with a towel. Allow mix to sit overnight.

3. Remix with the wire whisk, then package in powder cylinders.

GIFT IDEA

Decorate a powder cylinder with floral stickers or recycle a fluffy powder puff and pretty container. This makes a special gift for someone who is on her feet a lot.

LEMON RIND DEODORANT

This is a simple, natural way to stay fresh smelling and feeling.

Rind of 1 lemon

Yield: 1 treatment

To use:
Rub the fleshy side of the lemon rind under your armpits and allow to dry.

THYME AND ORANGE PEEL DEODORANT

More zesty than the Lemon Rind Deodorant, this is also a wonderful way to stay fresh.

¼ cup (50 ml) fresh thyme
Zest of 1 orange
½ cup (125 ml) apple cider vinegar

Yield: 4 ounces (100 g)

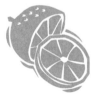

To make:
1. Place the fresh thyme and orange zest in a jar.
2. Pour the apple cider vinegar over the herbs and cover with a nonmetal lid.
3. Steep the mix for 2 weeks, shaking daily.
To use:
1. Pour 1 tablespoon (15 ml) of the vinegar over two cotton balls.
2. Rub the soaked cotton balls under each arm.

HERBS WITH DEODORIZING PROPERTIES

◆ Lemon juice
◆ Lovage
◆ Orange peel
◆ Orrisroot
◆ Patchouli
◆ Sagebrush
◆ Thyme
◆ Witch hazel

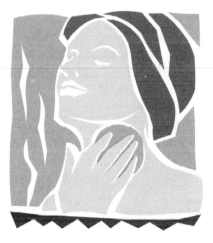

Skin Care for Sun Worshipers

CHAPTER 11

When skin is exposed to the sun, it produces melanin, which shows up as a suntan. Melanin acts to protect the skin from too much sun and from pollution. When you get a sunburn or stay in the sun too long during your first exposure, melanin will form quickly, but it will also peel. Repeated sunburns and overexposure to the sun increase the risk of skin cancer, especially for those with fair coloring.

Moderation, slow and gradual exposure, and sun protection can help shield your skin from the damaging effects. You may think that only commercial products can give you the sun protection you need, but in this chapter you'll find recipes for products that provide some sun protection, contain fewer chemicals than do commercial preparations, and offer various levels of moderate sun protection. If you have very fair skin, however, you may still want to purchase a product with a high sun protection factor (SPF).

While it is true that the sun provides the body with vitamin D, which helps build healthy bones, tanning depletes vitamin C and the B vitamins and also dehydrates the body. Keep this in mind during the summer especially, and eat a diet rich in these vitamins and water. Lots of fresh fruits and vegetables and eight 8-ounce glasses of water daily are recommended. Some people find vitamin supplements helpful. Deficiencies can result in patchy and blotchy skin and pigmentations.

SUN PROTECTION FORMULAS

The sun is necessary for health, but take care when you are outside. Unfortunately, the destruction of the ozone layer forces us to sun less or pay the consequences. In addition to being linked to skin cancer, overexposure to the sun breaks down collagen, the protein substance in the skin

---

WARNING SIGNS OF SKIN CANCER

Warning signs of skin cancer can often be seen in moles. Look for moles that have one or all of the following ABCs:

◆ Asymmetry
◆ Borders or edges that are irregular
◆ Color variations
◆ Diameter larger than the width of a pencil's eraser

Get in the habit of looking over your skin regularly; ask your partner to check your back. Any of these warning signs should be checked by a physician. Early detection is often key to a cure.

that gives it elasticity. The results are wrinkles, lines, and leathery-looking skin. I intentionally do not include a recipe here for tanning; you don't need me to tell you how to achieve that.

SUNSCREEN LOTION

Sesame oil offers the highest ultraviolet radiation absorption of any vegetable oil. The tannic acid in black tea also absorbs UV rays. Para-aminobenzoic acid (PABA), a B vitamin that you can purchase at your local pharmacy, is the main ingredient in commercial sunscreen products.

1 cup (250 ml) water
3 tea bags black tea
½ teaspoon (2 ml) PABA powder
2 tablespoons (30 ml) beeswax
1 cup (250 ml) sesame oil
10 drops vitamin E oil

Yield: 2 cups (500 ml)

To make:

1. Heat the water to boiling.

2. Place the tea bags in an 8- or 10-ounce (227- or 284-gram) jar.

3. Pour the boiling water over the tea bags, then cover the jar. Allow to steep until cooled to room temperature.

4. Remove the tea bags, pressing out all the water. Reserve the water. (Note: This will make the tea bitter, but you aren't going to drink it. The goal is to reserve the most tannic acid in the tea, which helps absorb ultraviolet rays.)

5. Dissolve the PABA powder into the tea.

6. In a double boiler, melt the beeswax in the sesame oil on low heat.

7. Once the beeswax is melted, remove from heat and allow to cool to room temperature.

8. Place the tea mixture in a blender on high speed. Slowly drizzle the oil mixture into it and mix for 5 minutes.

9. Add the vitamin E oil while still blending.

10. Pour into a clean container, preferably one with a spout.

To use:

1. Apply generously to your skin and face.

2. Reapply every 2 hours when the sun is hot and high.

ST.-JOHN'S-WORT OIL

St.-John's-wort oil repairs damage to the skin. The vermilion red oil is the preferred sunscreen of herbalists. It is also effective for treating sunburn and other burns. This oil can also be used as the oil portion of the moisturizer and cream recipes on pages 96 to 98.

2 cups (500 ml) flowering top of fresh St.-John's-wort herb

1 cup (250 ml) sesame oil

1 cup (250 ml) olive oil

10 drops vitamin E oil

Yield: 12 applications

To make:

1. Gather the St.-John's-wort midmorning when the top of the plant is flowering (July).
2. Spread the herb on paper towels and allow to wilt overnight.
3. The next day, stuff the herbs in a jar, packing it as full as possible.
4. Pour the oils over the herbs to fill the jar.
5. With a chopstick, poke the herbs, allowing them to release air and gases.
6. Top off with oil as necessary.
7. Store the oil in a dark, cool spot.
8. For the next 6 days, repeat steps 5, 6, and 7.
9. Let sit for the next 6 days, then on the 7th day repeat steps 5, 6, and 7.
10. Again, let sit for the next 6 days, then on the 7th day repeat steps 5, 6, and 7.
11. Let sit once more for the next 6 days, then strain the oil from the herbal material.
12. Add the vitamin E to the oil and store in an amber bottle.

To use:

1. Spread the oil lightly on all exposed areas.

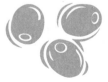

SUNBLOCK

Zinc oxide paste is a popular sunblock. Although I cannot tell you how to make neon-shaded cream naturally, this recipe goes on nicely and works as well as the more colorful commercial versions.

1 cup (250 ml) zinc oxide paste

½ cup (125 ml) sesame oil

½ cup (125 ml) orange blossom water, at room temperature

½ cup (125 ml) distilled water, at room temperature

Yield: 2 cups (500 ml)

To make:

1. Spoon the zinc oxide paste and pour the sesame oil into the top of a double boiler.

2. Stir as best you can. (It's sticky.)

3. Fill the bottom of the double boiler ¼ full of water and bring to a gentle boil.

4. Place the top of the pan containing the paste and oil over the bottom and gently heat, stirring constantly for 3 minutes.

5. Remove from heat. Add the orange blossom water and distilled water, mixing thoroughly.

6. Store in a widemouthed jar with lid; decorate with stickers, if desired.

To use:

1. Dab on the skin. Do not rub in. The more opaque the product is on you, the more effective the sunblock.

MOCK TAN

Just because you're protecting yourself from sunburn doesn't mean you can't have a bit of color. Henna, cloves, and black tea together offer a golden tan that looks like the real thing.

1 cup (250 ml) water
3 black tea bags
2 tablespoons (30 ml) whole cloves
2 cups (500 ml) brown henna or a henna that complements your skin tone
Clean, 2-inch-wide (5-cm) paintbrush

Yield: 1 full body treatment

To make:
1. Bring the water to a boil.
2. Place the tea bags in a jar that has a lid.
3. Pour the boiling water over the tea bags. Cap. Allow to steep for 20 minutes.
4. In a spice mill or coffee grinder, powder the cloves.
5. Strain the tea bags, reserving the tea.
6. Add the henna and powdered cloves to the tea.
7. Mix well to form a paste.

To use:
1. Standing on a plastic sheet, paint your body with a thin coat of paste, avoiding streaky lines.
2. Allow to dry and set for 10 minutes.
3. Shower as usual.

SOOTHING LOTIONS

These lotions ease the sting of sunburns, refresh in hot weather, and also relieve "the itches."

COOLING LOTION

So now you have a sunburn. The last thing you need is my preaching about the dangers of letting that happen! Here's a nourishing and cooling recipe that will take your pain away. (Try the Cucumber Body Pizza recipe found in chapter 7 for another cooling treatment.)

1 cup (250 ml) aloe vera gel
8 drops blue chamomile essential oil
20 drops vitamin E oil

Yield: 8 applications

To make:
1. Add the blue chamomile essential oil and vitamin E oil to the aloe vera gel.
2. Pour all ingredients into an amber bottle and shake well.
3. Store in the refrigerator.
To use:
Apply lightly to sunburned areas. This lotion also works well on other burns.

SUNBURN LOTION

This creamy lotion is soothing to sore skin, and moisturizing at the same time. It can be made with dried herbs, halving the quantity, but is better made from fresh ingredients.

¼ cup (50 ml) fresh chamomile

¼ cup (50 ml) fresh roses

¼ cup (50 ml) fresh comfrey

¼ cup (50 ml) fresh lavender

¼ cup (50 ml) fresh calendula

2 cups (500 ml) almond oil

¼ cup (50 ml) cocoa butter

⅔ cup (150 ml) coconut oil

Yield: 3 cups (750 ml)

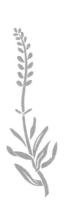

To make:

1. Gather the herbs in midmorning.

2. Spread the herbs on paper towels and allow them to wilt overnight.

3. The next day, stuff the herbs into a glass jar, packing it as full as possible.

4. Pour the almond oil over the herbs.

5. With a chopstick, poke the herbs to release air and gases.

6. Top off with oil as necessary to keep the herbs covered.

7. Store the oil in a dark, cool spot.

8. For each of the next six days, repeat steps 5, 6, and 7.

9. Let sit again for the next six days; on the seventh day, repeat steps 5, 6, and 7.

10. Again, let sit for six days; on the seventh day, repeat steps 5, 6, and 7.

11. Let sit for the next six days, then strain the oil from the herbal material.

12. In a double boiler, combine the cocoa butter and coconut oil with the herbal oil. Warm until all ingredients melt together.

13. Pour into a clean bottle, preferably one with a wide spout.

To use:

1. Shake well.

2. Pour the lotion in one hand and warm it by rubbing your hands together.

3. Apply to affected areas, or use all over as a moisturizer.

Storage:

Store in the refrigerator unless using often. To use, allow to warm fully and shake well.

LEMON LIGHTENING CREAM

This cream helps fade freckles, age spots, and the mask of pregnancy. The mask of pregnancy, also known as melasma, consists of brown patches that occur when women are pregnant, using birth-control pills, or, occasionally, for no specific reason. Pigmentation that occurs on women's skin may be attributable to elevated hormone levels, deficiencies in folic acid and other B vitamins, or picking and scratching. Protecting your skin from the sun is essential in fading the dark spots.

1/3 cup (75 ml) sesame oil
1/3 cup (75 ml) wheat germ oil
1/3 cup (75 ml) coconut oil
1 teaspoon (5 ml) cocoa butter
1 tablespoon (15 ml) beeswax
1 teaspoon (5 ml) alkanet root
3 tablespoons (45 ml) dried calendula
1/2 teaspoon (2 ml) folic acid powder
1/2 teaspoon (2 ml) PABA powder
2/3 cup (150 ml) distilled water
2 tablespoons (30 ml) lemon juice
1/3 cup (75 ml) aloe vera gel
10 drops vitamin E oil
10 drops lemon essential oil

Yield: 15 1-ounce (25-gram) jars

To make:

1. In a double boiler, heat the sesame, wheat germ, and coconut oils; cocoa butter; beeswax; alkanet root; and calendula flowers.

2. Once the beeswax is melted, strain out the alkanet root. Pour the oil mixture into a glass measuring cup, preferably one with a spout.

3. Let cool to room temperature for approximately 1 hour.

4. Set up your 15 clean 1-ounce (25-gram) jars on the edge of your counter for easy pouring.

5. Combine folic acid and PABA powder with the distilled water, lemon juice, aloe vera gel, vitamin E, and essential oil in the blender and turn to the highest speed for a minute or two.

6. Pour the cooled oils in a slow, thin drizzle into the vortex of the waters while the blender is still going.

7. Listen to the blender; when it chokes, the water and oil have combined.

8. Pour into the jars and decorate with stickers and ribbons.

Store containers in a cool place or refrigerate until ready to use.

ELBOW AND KNEE FADE TREATMENT

Do your knees and elbows get noticeably darker than the rest of your arms and legs? This recipe helps bleach the elbows and knees while exfoliating at the same time.

2 lemons
½ cup (125 ml) buttermilk
Paintbrush 1 inch (25 mm) wide
Gauze, enough to wrap both knees

Yield: 1 treatment for elbows and knees

To make:

1. Cut lemons in half and juice, saving the rinds.

2. Mix the lemon juice with the buttermilk.

To use:

1. Using a clean paintbrush, paint a thin coat of the lemon/buttermilk mixture on your knees.

2. Butterfly-cut the lemon rinds open (i.e., cut lemon in half, then cut again, leaving both quarters attached).

3. Spread a tablespoon of the mixture in each of the lemon half rinds and place two of them on your knees.

4. Wrap the gauze loosely around the knees and rinds, keeping them in the right place.

5. Paint a thin coat of the lemon/buttermilk mixture on your elbows.

6. Place a tablespoon of the lemon/buttermilk mixture in the remaining two lemon rinds.

7. Sit your elbows in the rinds.

8. Relax, leaving on for at least 20 minutes.

9. Rinse with tepid water.

PIGMENTATION PROBLEMS

If you have a lot of pigmention, you may want to check with your doctor or dermatologist about the possibility of supplementing your diet with B vitamins. You can do this by changing your eating habits to include more fresh fruits and vegetables, especially leafy greens, whole grains, mushrooms, molasses, liver, nutritional yeast, and wheat germ.

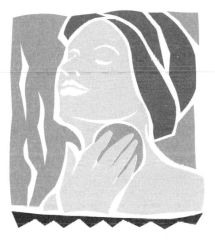

Putting It
All Together

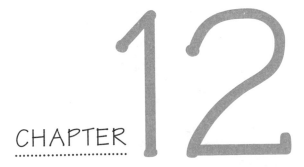

CHAPTER 12

It is easy enough to use the recipes in this book on an occasional basis — trying a recipe here and there as you get a chance or as a particular need or desire arises. That's great, but I encourage you to incorporate some of the treatments into your daily self-care routine. You will achieve the best results and the greatest benefit to your body if you give yourself these treatments on a regular basis. Following are suggestions for treatment combinations that you could use to develop an ongoing nurturing program. I also give suggestions for bringing together a group of friends for this purpose.

ESTABLISH A NEW TRADITION

When I was a child, my mother had her card parties. Why not start a tradition of nurturing parties? Maybe you already attend a women's group or a men's group: A few of the treatments could be the focus for a program or even an ongoing focus. Garden clubs that want a creative way to use their harvest can institute programs when herbs and flowers are bountiful.

Schedule Regular Appointments for Yourself

The most important part of any beauty ritual is making the time for it. It is easy for women to put themselves last, scheduling their lives around others. To really be of service to those in your life, you must take time for yourself. It demonstrates to your children the importance of spending time enhancing self-esteem. So get out your calendar. Schedule some treatments, and keep your appointments. You will feel better, and your family will benefit from your greater feelings of fulfillment because you put aside time for yourself.

A Chance to Share with Others

Many of the treatment combinations suggested in the following section are similar to those you might find at a resort or day spa. Take this opportunity to share time with your partner or another loved one so you can really enjoy yourself. These treatment combinations make a great gift for a special occasion, such as a birthday, anniversary, or job promotion.

Herbal home spa treatments also offer a nice chance to share an activity with your children, especially daughters. Children love to make some of the easier recipes (e.g., lip balm, soap balls, henna tattoos, or nail color) that they can use themselves and give to their friends as gifts. Children can also learn to give and receive nurturing treatments. A massage is a great chance for you to nurture each other and share the loving touch.

SUGGESTED TREATMENT ROUTINES

You probably already have daily morning and evening cleansing routines. You may be surprised at how little effort it takes to substitute nourishing herbal body treatments for your more conventional ones, and how much better they will make you feel about yourself and your body.

Daily Treatments

In the morning:

◆ Use an all-over skin exfoliation technique such as Roman Skin Brushing, Ayate Fiber Rub, Loofah Scrub, or Garshan Silk Mitt Treatment.

◆ Cleanse your face using an herbal cleansing milk or gel.

◆ Tone skin using floral water or herbal astringent.

◆ Apply Violet Eye Cream.

◆ Apply nail oil or cream.

◆ Massage in a facial cream with sun protection.

In the evening:

◆ Use an all-over skin exfoliation technique such as Roman Skin Brushing, Ayate Fiber Rub, Loofah Scrub, or Garshan Silk Mitt Treatment.

◆ Cleanse face with avena cleansing grains.

◆ Tone skin using floral water or an herbal astringent.

Weekly Treatments

◆ Herbal facial steam or Papaya Enzyme Treatment

◆ Oxygen Facial or Peel-off Mask

◆ Herbal body scrub

◆ Herbal bath treatment

◆ Scalp treatment

◆ Herbal hair rinse

DON'T MOISTURIZE AT NIGHT

Contrary to many skin-care programs, I do not recommend using a moisturizer or night cream on your skin before bed. My experience is that a natural detoxification occurs at night. This process brings the natural oils of the face to the surface, allowing the skin to circulate, breath, and naturally moisturize itself. The use of creams at night blocks these processes.

Monthly Treatments

- ◆ Herbal foot scrub and bath
- ◆ Herbal body wrap
- ◆ Infused oil massage

PLANNING A DAY OF BEAUTY IN YOUR HERBAL HOME SPA

Once you've got your home spa up and running and you've tried some of the treatments, make an appointment for yourself to enjoy a day of beauty there. For best results, prepare as much as you can a day in advance, so you can just sit back and enjoy the treatment. It is also nice to make a special light lunch and have some brewed herbal tea ready so you can enjoy yourself without any work on this relaxing day. Do the treatments in the order suggested here.

HERBAL HOME SPA TREATMENT PROGRAMS

Full-Day Program One	Full-Day Program Two	Half-Day Program
Roman Dry Brushing	Flower Essence Scalp Massage	Ayate Fiber Rub
Oatmeal Almond Body Scrub	Violet Eye Cream	Seaweed Body Wrap
Rose Petal Vinegar Bath	Herbal Facial Steam	Papaya Enzyme Facial Treatment
Cucumber Eye Pack	Peel-off Mask	Deep Pore Treatment
Oxygen Facial	Floral Water	Queen of Hungary Water
Paraffin Hand and Foot Treatment	Garshan Silk Mitt Treatment	Lip Balm
Creamy Lotion Full-body Massage	Cellulite Body Wrap	Lavender Blue Face Moisturizer
	Hot and Cold Stimulation	
	Rose Pink Face Moisturizer	

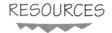
PUBLICATIONS

Herbal Gram
P.O. Box 201660
Austin, TX 78720
Magazine

The Herb Quarterly
P.O. Box 689
San Anselmo, CA 94960
Magazine

Interweave Press
The Herb Companion
201 East Fourth Street
Loveland, CO 80537

EDUCATIONAL ORGANIZATIONS

American Botanical Council
P.O. Box 201660
Austin, TX 78720
(512) 331-8868

**American Herbal Products
Association**
P.O. Box 2410
Austin, TX 78768
(512) 320-8555

American Herb Association
P.O. Box 1673
Nevada City, CA 95959
(916) 265-9552 (FAX)

Greta's Garden Herb School
763 Route 295
East Chatham, NY 12060
518-392-7245
*Offers classes and workshops on a
variety of herbal and country arts
topics, including medicinal appren-
ticeships, herbal skin care, and culinary herbs. Herbal-product catalog.*

**Herb Growing & Marketing
Network**
P.O. Box 245
Silver Spring, PA 17575

Herb Research Foundation
1007 Pearl St. Suite 200
Boulder, CO 80802
(303) 449-2265

Northeast Herbal Association
P.O. Box 479
Milton, NY 12547

United Plant Savers
P.O. Box 420
East Barre, VT 05649
(802) 476-3722

MAIL-ORDER SOURCES

Atlantic Spice Company
P.O. Box 205
N. Truro, MA 02652
(800) 316-7965
Fax (508) 487-2550
Website: www.atlanticspice.com
Free herbal catalog.

Brushy Mountain Bee Farm
610 Bethany Church Road
Moravian Falls, NC 28654
(800) 233-7929
Fax (910) 921-2681
*Free catalog; hex jars, honey,
beeswax.*

Burch Bottle and Packaging
811 10th Street
Watervliet, NY 12189
(800) 903-2830
Fax (518) 273-1846

Dry Creek Herb Farm
13935 Dry Creek Road
Auburn, CA 95602
(916) 878-2441

Frontier Co-op Herbs
3021 78th Street
P.O. Box 299
Norway, IA 52318
(800) 669-3275
Fax (800) 717-4372
Website: www.frontierherb.com
Free herbal-supply catalog.

Green Terrestrial Herbal Products
P.O. Box 266
Milton, NY 12547
(914) 795-5238

Janca's Jojoba
456 E. Juanita #7
Mesa, AZ 85204
(602) 496-9494
Fax (602) 479-1312
Free catalog; oils, cosmetic ingredients.

Lavender Lane
7337 #1 Roseville Road
Sacramento, CA 95842
(888) 593-4400
Fax (916) 339-0842
Free catalog.

Liberty Natural Products
8120 SE Stark Street
Portland, OR 97215
(503) 256-1227

Margaret's Magicals
P.O. Box 846
Planetarian Station
New York, NY 10024-0540
(212) 496-6726

Mountain Rose Herbs
20818 High Street
North San Juan, CA 95960
(800) 879-3337
Fax (916) 292-9138
Organically grown herbs, cosmetic ingredients, bottles.

Naomi's Herbs
11 Housatonic Street
Lenox, MA 01240
(888) 462-6647

Norfolk Lavender
2031 Rte. 130
Monmouths Junction, NJ 08852
(800) 886-0050
Fax (732) 422-2290

Once Upon a Thyme
3606 State Route 22
85 Battenkill Evergreens
Salem, NY 12865
(518) 854-7924
Catalog; specializes in herb plants.

Presque Isle Wine Cellars
9440 West Main
Northeast, PA 16428
(814) 725-1314
Free catalog; bottle cuffs, finishing touches for vinegars, etc.

Sunburst Bottle
5710 Auburn Boulevard #7
Sacramento, CA 95841
(916) 348-5576
Fax (800) 810-0440

Vermont Country Store
P.O. Box 3000
Manchester Center, VT 05255-3000
(802) 362-2400
Fax (802) 362-0285

BIBLIOGRAPHY

Cavitch, Susan Miller. *The Natural Soap Book.* Pownal, VT: Storey Communications, Inc., 1995.

Cox, Janice. *Natural Beauty at Home.* New York: Henry Holt and Company, 1995.

Dincin Buchman, Dian. *The Complete Herbal Guide to Natural Health and Beauty.* New Canaan, CT: Keats Publishing, 1973.

Dodt, Colleen K. *The Essential Oils Book.* Pownal, VT: Storey Communications, Inc., 1996.

Facetti, Aldo. *Natural Beauty.* New York: Simon and Schuster Inc., 1990.

Gladstar, Rosemary. *Herbal Healing for Women.* New York: Fireside, 1993.

———. *Natural Cosmetics and Skin Care.* East Barre, VT: Sage, n.d.

Hampton, Aubrey. *Natural Organic Hair and Skin Care.* Tampa, FL: Organica Press, 1987.

Harris, Jessica. *The World Beauty Book.* San Francisco: HarperCollins, 1995.

Hoffman, David. *The New Holistic Herbal.* Rockport, MA: Element, Inc., 1992.

Kanner, Catherine. *Beauty from a Country Garden.* Berkeley, CA: Ten Speed Press, 1992.

Kloss, Jethro. *Back to Eden.* Santa Barbara, CA: Lifeline Books, 1972.

Krochmal, Connie. *Natural Cosmetics from Beehive to Herb Garden.* Moravian Falls, NC: Brushy Mountain Bee Farm, n.d.

Magic and Medicine of Plants. Pleasantville, NY: Reader's Digest, Inc., 1986.

McClure, Susan. *The Herb Gardener.* Pownal, VT: Storey Communications, Inc., 1997.

Norman, Laura. *Feet First: A Guide to Foot Reflexology.* New York: Fireside, 1988.

Rose, Jeanne. *Herbs and Things.* New York: Perigee Books, 1972.

———. *Jeanne Rose's Herbal Body Book.* New York: Perigee Books, 1976.

———. *Kitchen Cosmetics.* Berkeley, CA: North Atlantic Books, 1978.

Tourles, Stephanie. *The Herbal Body Book.* Pownal, VT: Storey Communications, Inc., 1995.

Pattern for Cover

Pattern for Herbal Eye Pillow

(increase pattern on photocopier by 25%)

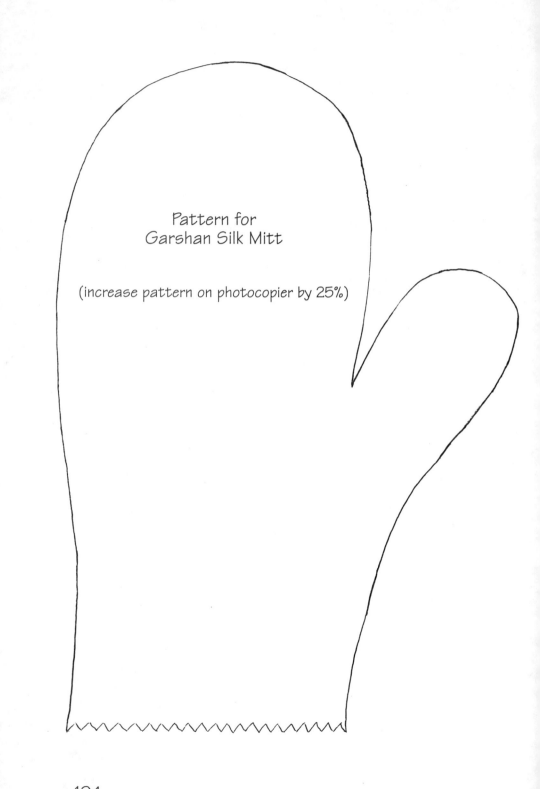

Pattern for
Garshan Silk Mitt

(increase pattern on photocopier by 25%)

INDEX

Page references in *italics* indicate illustrations;
those in **bold** indicate charts.

The Herbal Home Remedy Book: Simple Recipes for Tinctures, Teas, Salves, Tonics, and Syrups, by Joyce A. Wardwell. Enables the reader to identify and use twenty-five easy-to-find herbs to make simple remedies in the form of teas, tinctures, salves, tonics, vinegars, syrups, and lozenges. Gives hundreds of suggestions for maintaining health and well-being simply, naturally, and inexpensively. Folklore — including Native American legends and stories — provides information on the origins of many herbal medicines. 176 pages. Paperback. ISBN -58017-016-1.

The Herbal Body Book: A Natural Approach to Healthier Hair, Skin, and Nails, by Stephanie Tourles. Contains more than 100 recipes to transform common herbs, fruits, and grains into safe, economical, and natural personal care items such as facial scrubs, shampoos, lip balms, powders, and more. 128 pages. Paperback. ISBN 0-88266-880-3.

The Essential Oils Book: Creating Personal Blends for Mind and Body, by Colleen K. Dodt. Discusses the many uses of aromatherapy and its applications in everyday life. Includes simple recipes that anyone can make from ingredients available at health food stores or herb shops. 160 pages. Paperback. ISBN 0-88266-913-3.

Natural BabyCare: Pure and Soothing Recipes and Techniques for Mothers and Babies, by Colleen K. Dodt. Offers recipes for creating natural personal care items for babies, such as lotions, bath and massage oils, creams, shampoos, powders, and more. Also features self-care during pregnancy and childbirth. 160 pages. Paperback. ISBN 0-88266-953-2.

The Natural Soap Book: Making Herbal and Vegetable-Based Soaps, by Susan Miller Cavitch. Provides basic vegetable-based soap recipes along with ideas on scenting, coloring, trimming, and wrapping soaps. 192 pages. Paperback. ISBN 0-88266-888-9.

Milk-Based Soaps: Making Natural, Skin-Nourishing Soap, by Casey Makela. Foolproof instructions for creating twelve distinctive soaps, all suitable for either goat's or cow's milk. 112 pages. Paperback. ISBN 0-88266-984-2.

Perfumes, Splashes & Colognes: Discovering and Crafting Your Personal Fragrances, by Nancy M. Booth. Profiles basic scent and perfume ingredients, and offers recipes for creating personalized scents or recreating popular perfumes at a fraction of the cost of the original. 176 pages. Paperback. ISBN 0-88266-985-0.

*These books and other Storey books are available
at your bookstore, farm store, garden center, or directly from
Storey Books, Schoolhouse Road, Pownal, Vermont 05261,
or by calling 800-441-5700. Visit our Web site at www.storey.com.*